The Mindfulness Prescription for Adult ADHD

The Mindfulness Prescription for

Adult ADHD

An Eight-Step Program for
Strengthening Attention,
Managing Emotions, and
Achieving Your Goals

LIDIA ZYLOWSKA, MD

Foreword by Daniel J. Siegel, MD

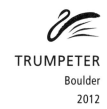

TRUMPETER
Boulder
2012

Trumpeter Books
An imprint of Shambhala Publications, Inc.
4720 Walnut Street
Boulder, Colorado 80301
www.shambhala.com

Photos on pages 45–46 showing meditation posture reprinted courtesy of the Mountains and Rivers Order National Buddhist Archives.

The emotion categories on pages 152–53 are reprinted with permission from the collaborative database on emotion-related language for technological contexts. Accessed from http://emotion-research.net/projects/humaine/earl/proposal#Categories.

The World Health Organization Adult ADHD Self-Report Scale (ASRS-v1.1) Symptom Checklist on pages 206–7 is reprinted with permission.

14 13 12 11 10 9 8 7 6

Printed in the United States of America

♾ This edition is printed on acid-free paper that meets the American National Standards Institute Z39.48 Standard.

♻ This book is printed on 30% postconsumer recycled paper. For more information please visit www.shambhala.com.

Distributed in the United States by Penguin Random House LLC and in Canada by Random House of Canada Ltd

Interior design and composition by Greta D. Sibley

Library of Congress Cataloging-in-Publication Data
Zylowska, Lidia.
The mindfulness prescription for adult ADHD: an 8-step program for strengthening attention, managing emotions, and achieving your goals / Lidia Zylowska; foreword by Daniel Siegel.
p.   cm.
ISBN 978-1-59030-847-9 (pbk.)
1. Attention-deficit disorder in adults—Alternative treatment—Popular works.
2. Attention-deficit hyperactivity disorder—Popular works. 3. Mind and body therapies—Popular works. 4. Self-care, Health—Popular works. I. Title.
RC394.A85Z95 2012
616.85'89—dc23
2011025174

To the memory of my father, Jozef Zylowski

Contents

Foreword   ix

Acknowledgments   xiii

Prologue   xv

Dear Reader
Do Something Different This Time   1

Part 1 **MINDFULNESS**
You Can Train Your Mind

1. A Different Way of Paying Attention   11

2. Mindfulness and Self-Regulation in ADHD   23

3. Getting Ready for the Eight-Step Program   43

Part 2 **MINDFULNESS FOR ADHD**
The Eight-Step Program

Introduction   53

STEP 1. Become More Present
Attention and the Five Senses   55

STEP 2. Focus the Wandering Mind
         Mindful Breathing   69

STEP 3. Direct and Anchor Your Awareness
         Mindfulness of Sound, Breath, and Body   80

STEP 4. Listen to Your Body
         Mindfulness of Body Sensations and Movement   89

STEP 5. Observe Your Mind
         Mindfulness of Thoughts   110

STEP 6. Manage Your Emotions
         Mindfulness of Feelings   128

STEP 7. Communicate Skillfully
         Mindful Listening and Speaking   154

STEP 8. Slow Down to Be More Effective
         Mindful Decisions and Actions   169

    4.   Putting It All Together
         Using Mindfulness in Your Daily Life with ADHD   194

         Frequently Asked Questions (FAQ)   202

         ADHD Symptoms Checklist   206

         List of Mindfulness Exercises   209

         Notes   211

         Index   221

         About the Author   229

         CD Track List   230

Foreword

Daniel J. Siegel, MD

In your hands you have a practical approach to helping you focus attention, balance your emotions, improve your relationships, and enhance your life. Sounds too good to be true, doesn't it? Well, research supports the suggestions made in this book: The way you focus your mind can actually change the structure of your brain. No kidding. By taking the practical steps in this book, you can strengthen the connections in your brain that support a more focused way of living. People with and even without ADHD can benefit from learning to develop mindful awareness in their lives. This book is tailored for those with attentional challenges, who will find it especially relevant and accessible to use.

But why would it help to be "mindful" or to learn to have "mindful awareness"? Think of it this way: Our attention is the way energy flows through us. Sometimes we can focus that energy, say, into listening to what someone is saying to us. But then a radio program catches our ear or a television screen catches our eye, and the words of our friend are far from the focus of our attention. Such distractions can make us lose our ability to remember what the other person was saying and they put stress on a relationship. Not so good! If that person is a friend, a spouse, a teacher, or a boss, such distractions can lead to big and lasting problems. We can feel bad, and the other person can feel disrespected. It's tough for everyone when attention is on the run. And for young people, being unable to focus attention can make challenges to creating a positive sense of who they are. It is hard to be told that you are not doing what you are supposed to do, and being told this over and over and over and over and over and over again. Enough is enough!

Now there is a new prescription to such challenges to ADHD, a practical approach that can be used alongside commonly prescribed medications, if they are being used. Lidia Zylowska, MD, headed up our pilot study at the UCLA Mindful Awareness Research Center. With our coworkers at the center, she created a mindfulness-based program that has a potential to dramatically improve focus and other "executive skills" in adults and adolescents with attentional difficulties. The lessons learned from this initial pilot study need to be confirmed through additional research, but the study's findings and Dr. Zylowska's clinical experience with her patients are offered here for you in this easy-to-use, readily accessible guide for those with ADHD.

What's in this for you? You can use these practical tools to transform your life. By learning to focus attention in a new way, you can actually strengthen the very brain areas that are creating challenges in focusing and maintaining attention. You'll also learn how to balance your emotions and create and nurture more rewarding relationships. It's amazing, but true. You don't have to be bullied by your brain's wandering focus anymore. Now you can actually befriend your brain by learning mindful skills of attention as practiced in the helpful exercises throughout this book.

Some people say, "If I was born with a genetic issue like ADHD, how could anything short of a pill help my brain?" What we can now say very clearly, based on mounting research, is that even those with inborn issues—like mood or anxiety or attention challenges—can learn to train their minds and thereby change their brains. The secret ingredient to these changes is training attention, which in these pages you'll learn how to do.

But why, you might ask, would attention change the brain? And how do we know this can happen? Attention is the focus of energy through the nervous system. When neurons—the basic cells of the brain—are firing off with attention, they actually alter their connections. When you learn a practice like being mindfully aware, you activate and then strengthen the executive circuits of the brain responsible for such things as attention, regulating emotions, being flexible in your responses, insightful, empathic, and even being wise. No fooling. We know this in general to be true from a wide set of studies of the brains of those who've learned to practice mindful awareness. Mindfulness practice involves the focus of attention—a focus that drives energy though the brain and strengthens it much like exercise strengthens a muscle. Mindful awareness training—the lessons of this book—builds up the muscle of the mind.

So why not give it a try? You have everything to gain and it just takes your willingness to say, "Let's go!" Dive in, learn a lot, and have fun.

Daniel J. Siegel, MD
Clinical Professor of Psychiatry, UCLA School of Medicine
Co-Director, UCLA Mindful Awareness Research Center
Executive Director, Mindsight Institute

Acknowledgments

I am grateful to a number of people who in diverse and generous ways have contributed to this book. First of all, I want to thank my editors at Trumpeter Books: Eden Steinberg, for her invaluable input throughout the writing process, and Ben Gleason, for shepherding the book to its publication. I am also thankful to Stephanie Tade for her support as my literary agent and Karalynn Ott for her early edits.

This book would not be possible without the contributions of many of my professional colleagues. I am greatly appreciative of Dr. Kenneth Wells, who mentored me throughout the UCLA Robert Wood Johnson Clinical Scholars Program. I am indebted to faculty of the UCLA Mindful Awareness Research Center, especially those who directly contributed to my research—namely, Dr. Susan Smalley, Diana Winston, and Dr. Deborah Ackerman—and to Dr. Daniel Siegel for his steadfast support throughout the years and his contribution of a foreword to this book.

I am grateful to other clinicians and mentors who have been instrumental in growing my understanding of mindfulness meditation: Dr. Ka Kit Hui for introducing me to mind-body medicine, Dr. James Finely for offering wonderful insights into mindfulness and encouragement in my work, and Dr. Jeffrey Schwartz for discussing with me his pioneering neuroscience-based approach to mindfulness. The writings and work of Dr. Jon Kabat-Zinn, Dr. Zindel Segal, Dr. Mark Williams, and Dr. John Teasdale provided a model for my work in ADHD, and I greatly admire them and other teachers of mindfulness for their compassionate work.

I thank my colleagues Dr. Mark Bertin, Mimi Handlin, Dr. Elisha Goldstein, and Dr. Ari Tuckman for their encouragement in writing this book; Dr. Edward Hallowell for his generous review; and my patients for sharing their stories with me.

The process of writing my first book was both challenging and rewarding, and I want to thank my mother and other family and friends for supporting me in many ways throughout this journey. You are the wise, kind, and loving presence in my life. In writing this book I am especially indebted to my sister Agnieszka and my brother-in-law Michael Goeller for their valuable reviews of my early ideas.

Thanks to my cat Boots, who was a wonderful reminder of the present moment as I wrote. Last, but most important, I want to thank my loving husband Jeff for being there in the trenches with me, keeping me fed and sane, and offering helpful comments on the book.

Prologue

Between stimulus and response there is a space.
In that space is our power to choose our response. In
our response lies our growth and our freedom.

—Viktor Frankl, *Man's Search for Meaning*

- If there were a mental training that improved your attention, impulse control, and quality of life—would you try it?
- If you could step back from old patterns and reactions and create a new way of handling stress and taking action in your life—would you do it?
- If you could have more emotional balance and ability for joy—would you be willing to make lifestyle changes?
- If you could be more present to yourself and your loved ones—would that inspire and motivate you?
- If you could have greater control over your ADHD symptoms—would that make a difference?
- If you could have greater appreciation for who you are, both with your ADHD and non-ADHD sides—would you be happier?

If you're intrigued by any or all of these questions, this book is for you. *The Mindfulness Prescription for Adult ADHD* will deepen your understanding of ADHD and provide a new set of tools and techniques for managing it.

Any change and growth starts with awareness. And while there are many ways to increase awareness — education, life experience, others' feedback — the ability to tune in to the present moment, where everything happens in real time, creates tremendous opportunities for change. Mindfulness is a training in such present-moment awareness, and this book describes how this type of training can help adults with ADHD.

As a psychiatrist specializing in adult ADHD and mindfulness-based therapies, I've helped many adults learn to manage their ADHD symptoms through mindfulness training. Mindfulness has been shown to be an effective approach to stress, anxiety, and depression, and it has positive effects on brain health. There is still much to learn about this powerful tool for ADHD, and I hope this book will ignite more interest in mindfulness across the ADHD field. I invite you to discover and explore this treatment with me.

The Mindfulness Prescription for Adult ADHD

Dear Reader,

Do Something Different This Time

If you're like me and often skip book introductions, I invite you to *do something different this time.*

I invite you to notice with curiosity any impulse you may feel to jump ahead, and yet please resist that impulse and read on. This introductory letter will give you a sense of where I am coming from and lay the groundwork for the rest of the book.

If you take the time to read this section, this could be your first opportunity to practice mindful awareness. You can notice your *habitual or automatic response* (in this case, to not read the introduction), and you can explore having a *new sense of awareness and choice about your actions.*

If, on the other hand, you're the type of person who usually reads introductions, I encourage you to read on with the enhanced awareness that *not* skipping the introduction this time is not just your habit, but it is also a deliberate choice.

So, first things first. This book is for those who have, or think they may have, attention deficit hyperactivity disorder, or ADHD. The common abbreviation *ADD* is another casual and popular way to refer to ADHD, especially ADHD without hyperactivity, but in general, *ADHD* is a more precise, scientifically recognized term that refers to *all* the types of this condition (for example, ADHD-inattentive, ADHD-hyperactive, or ADHD-combined subtypes). For simplicity's sake, I'll use the term ADHD through-out the book when talking about all types of the condition.

Following is a quick checklist of common ADHD difficulties.

❑ Do you have trouble paying attention and are you easily bored or distracted?
❑ Is it hard for you to get organized?
❑ Do you have trouble starting or finishing projects?
❑ Do you dread paperwork and have trouble keeping up with your mail?
❑ Do you frequently lose or misplace important items such as your keys or your wallet?
❑ Are you often late paying your bills and so charged with extra fees?
❑ Do you frequently feel restless, have trouble relaxing, and find that you have to keep busy all the time?
❑ Do you tend to change jobs more than others or have "too many interests"?
❑ Do you interrupt others when they are speaking or blurt things out even when you don't want to?
❑ Is it hard for you to manage your time well or not be chronically late?
❑ Are you often bored, impatient, easily frustrated, or have trouble with emotional ups and downs?

If you answered "yes" to most of these questions, you may be an adult with ADHD. If you haven't been diagnosed by a professional, please bring this up with your primary care doctor, therapist, or, preferably, with an ADHD specialist. This condition, often associated with children, can also affect adults. We now know that at least 50 percent of children with ADHD continue to have difficulties as adults, and in the United States 4 percent or more of the total adult population report significant ADHD symptoms.

While we all can feel spacey, restless, or forgetful at times, adults with ADHD struggle with these feelings *most* of the time. If you have ADHD, problems with unruly attention, disorganization, restlessness, impulsivity, and intense emotions can create a lot of difficulties in your life and can stop you from reaching your full potential in school, at work, and in relationships. These problems are not just an occasional nuisance or frustration—they are frequent occurrences that can give you a chronic sense of not being able to rely on yourself.

Overall, ADHD leads to difficulties with self-control, or what professionals call *self-regulation*. Here is an example: One minute you may be getting ready to leave home for a job interview, but an incoming e-mail grabs your attention. You then start reading all of your e-mail and lose track of time, only to realize that now you're late for the appointment. You berate yourself for getting distracted and feel panicked about getting going. Feeling frazzled, you rush out the door without your résumé! The whole day becomes highly stressful as you try to make it to the meeting, even though it's already too late. This ADHD cycle can repeat itself over and over again, leading to chronic stress, self-doubt, and ever-increasing difficulty getting things done and reaching your goals.

Since ADHD interferes with the development of a person's self-control, tools and techniques that improve self-regulation can be of great help. *Mindfulness or mindful awareness*—a type of mental training derived from meditation practices—is one such tool. This book invites you to explore mindfulness as a way to understand and manage the symptoms of adult ADHD.

Try It for Yourself

Let's do a quick experiment. Can you turn your attention to the experience of holding this book right now? Shift your attention to your present-moment sensations. If you are sitting, notice how your body makes contact with the chair. Do you notice any points of pressure or weight? If you are standing, for example on a crowded bus or subway, notice your body posture. Now shift your attention to your feet. Notice any sensations such as tingling or pressure in your feet. Perhaps you notice a lack of sensation. After a few moments, shift your attention to your hands. What are your hands doing right now? Notice the point of contact with the book and how it feels to be touching the paper.

....

The essence of mindfulness is intentionally bringing your attention to the present moment with openness and curiosity.

....

Mindfulness puts you in the driver's seat, directing your attention where you want it to go. Much of our daily experience is just the other way around. Our attention is often pulled in many directions, or we are lost in thought, preoccupied. Multitasking, the scores of demands at home and work, and constant e-mail messages or phone calls create a slew of opportunities for distraction. After all, as people say, we live in an "ADD culture," and even many people who don't actually have ADHD feel they can't concentrate. If you have ADHD, the pitfalls of such distracting environments are magnified, since your attention naturally tends to jump from one thing to another.

Mindfulness (or mindful awareness) is the opposite of being distracted, lost in thought, or daydreaming. Mindfulness is about being alert and aware of what we are doing as we are doing it. It involves tracking our experience moment by moment to see clearly and simply what *is*—without being limited by automatic responses, judgments, and expectations. Mindfulness brings awareness, reflection, and choice—and is the opposite of being on autopilot.

At its core, mindfulness embraces heartfulness, as it requires being kind and compassionate to yourself and your experiences. So often we end up criticizing ourselves for how we are or what we feel, and that stops us from learning from our experiences. This judgmental or hypercritical perspective can leave us stuck, ashamed, or hypersensitive. It can also lead us to pretend nothing is wrong with our behavior, when we know full well that something is amiss. Mindfulness helps us accept ourselves as we are right now and, paradoxically, through acceptance, leads to possibilities for growth and change.

Mindfulness = Heartfulness

The practice of mindfulness, derived from meditation, is a way to strengthen your attention skills, develop self-awareness, and improve your emotional well-being. It is a type of mental training that can be done in many different ways, with or without formal meditation—great news for those of us who, like me, have trouble sitting still for a long time!

Increasingly, mindfulness is being successfully used as a treatment for physical and mental problems such as chronic pain, stress, depression, anxiety, and addictions. Studies conducted at academic centers around the world over the past several years are showing that after an eight-week training in mindfulness, different groups of people, ranging from medical students to patients with depression to elementary school children, show improvements in mental health symptoms and a greater sense of well-being.[1] Studies in neuroscience, meanwhile, point to the ability of mental exercises such as mindfulness to enhance the brain circuits responsible for attention and emotion regulation.[2]

My Introduction to Mindfulness

I first learned about mindfulness in the late 1990s during my psychiatry residency at the University of California–Los Angeles (UCLA). Curious about using complementary and alternative medicines for psychiatry, I decided to do a fellowship at the UCLA Center for East-West Medicine. While there I was exposed to mind-body practices, including meditation. I learned about existing programs like Mindfulness-Based Stress Reduction and Mindfulness-Based Cognitive Therapy, and I quickly became fascinated with the power of mindfulness training both for myself and my patients. I read all I could about it and then started attending mindfulness workshops or training sessions, where I got to experience the mindful awareness firsthand. It was transforming.

My big epiphany came when I realized I could *pay attention to my attention*. I learned that I could observe my thoughts, feelings, or body responses in a new way, without being caught up in them or without wanting to change them. At my first week-long meditation retreat, I experienced brief moments of observing my busy mind in an entirely different way—by witnessing it rather than being controlled by it. At one point, I noticed that upsetting feelings began bubbling up inside me, but rather than pushing them away or being completely overwhelmed, I chose to pay attention to how my body felt when I was really upset. That's when I realized that my thoughts were often judgmental or unkind to myself or others, and I discovered that the introduction of gentleness and kindness allowed me to learn about the places where I was "stuck."

I also realized how hard it is to keep mindfulness practice consistent in my life, despite my best intentions. As with physical exercise, knowing that it is good for me is not always enough to get me to do it! So I learned to bring moments of mindfulness into my life as much as I could throughout the day, even if for just one breath.

My own experience with mindfulness taught me that its practice is a powerful and important tool for psychological well-being, and I wanted to study how it could be applied to adults who struggle with ADHD. In 2004 I led the creation of a program called Mindful Awareness Practices (MAPs) for ADHD at UCLA's Mindful Awareness Research Center. The MAPs program teaches how to strengthen attention, balance emotions, and manage life with ADHD.

Our initial study tested this program with a group of adults and teens with ADHD.[3] The eight-week training was well received, and we found that it made a significant positive difference in how participants experienced their ADHD symptoms and their well-being. Afterward, a majority of the participants reported decreased ADHD symptoms as well as less anxiety, depression, and stress. Most of them also performed better on selected cognitive tests that measured different aspects of attention, memory, and reasoning. In particular they appeared to have had an enhanced ability to pay attention under distracting conditions.

One participant in our study told us, "I understand better what goes on in my head, and I'm less critical of myself which is a positive result from the class.... I'm less reactive and I'm more forgiving of myself." Another said, "The idea that you can see yourself getting distracted and then you can bring yourself back was probably the most pivotal thing.... And the experience of practicing it in the meditation—going off and then coming back. So, when I'm aware now that I'm distracting myself from a task, I'm able to see it better and then get back a little better."

This initial study did not have a control group, and more studies are needed to confirm the positive effects of mindfulness training on ADHD symptoms, but the research is building. Recently, Anna Uliando and her colleagues at Deakin University in Australia have adapted the MAPs program to eight-to-twelve-year olds with ADHD. In a well-designed, controlled study, fifteen children enrolled in the eight-week program, and they were compared to twenty children who did ADHD "treatment as usual." The overall results (as yet unpublished) supported the findings of our study with teens and adults: mindfulness training led to improvements in certain aspects of attention, ADHD symptoms, anxiety, and depression.

Over the last several years, I have also used mindfulness in my clinical practice with many adults with ADHD. This book is based on my work with patients and includes many of their stories and experiences.*

---

*Patients' names have been changed to protect their confidentiality.

How This Book Is Organized

Part 1 of the book describes mindfulness in more detail and shows how this approach can help those with ADHD. In part 2, the core of the book, I present mindfulness training as a series of eight sequential steps that can be done over a period of eight weeks; however, feel free to proceed at your own pace. An audio CD is included with this book to guide you through the key mindfulness practices. (The audio program is also available as a free audio download at www.shambhala.com/MindfulnessPrescription.) The concluding chapter of the book discusses how to use mindfulness in daily life with ADHD and answers frequently asked questions. An index of mindfulness practices and additional resources are available in the backmatter.

If you have ADHD it may be easier for you to learn information when it's presented in a quick, "bullet point" way without lengthy explanations. In general, I've found that images, stories, or text boxes (such as sidebars) often help those with ADHD to read more easily and understand the main points of a reading. And so, this book will:

- Introduce mindfulness as a helpful tool for adults with ADHD and their families.
- Show how you can use mindfulness to neutralize the negative effects of ADHD symptoms and to thrive despite having ADHD.
- Present the information in an ADHD-friendly, easy-to-learn way.

My hope is that this book will engender your curiosity about different ways you can attend to and relate to all your daily experiences. I also hope that you'll continue learning about mindfulness throughout your life, make it your own, and keep exploring your inner resources for insight, self-compassion, and positive action. As you explore mindfulness, feel free to let me know what you discover.

Best wishes on your mindful ADHD journey!

Dr. Z

Part One

MINDFULNESS

You Can Train Your Mind

1 A Different Way of Paying Attention

My experience is what I agree to attend to.
—William James, *The Principles of Psychology*

Attention is our window to the world, both the world outside of us and the world within. It is attention that allows certain information to stream in and become part of our conscious experience. The decision to give something attention determines what we see and don't see, what we are aware of and what we miss. As attention shapes our awareness, it informs our choices and our actions, and—as we now know from neuroscience research—attention also shapes the function and the structure of our brains. Ultimately, where we place our attention, and how other things grab our attention, shapes our lives.

Where we place our attention shapes our lives.

Believe it or not, the power of attention to determine our lives is not bad news for people with ADHD. It's true that underlying genetics often make it hard for those with ADHD to control their attention. But that's not the whole story. Whether or not you have ADHD, you still have the ability to direct your attention at will and develop greater awareness of your responses. The scientific research on attention shows that this mental quality can be trained in both children and in adults—and in those with attention deficits and those without them. So the good news is that even if you do have ADHD, you can train and strengthen your attention to become more empowered to work with your ADHD symptoms.

But how is attention and awareness trained? Since the late 1990s, computer programs have been developed to strengthen attention and memory in ADHD, and they show some promise.[1] More work is needed, however, to confirm these benefits and understand how they affect the whole person: their emotions, behavior, and interaction in the real world. And while new brain-training technology is being investigated, Eastern meditative traditions such as Buddhism also offer a way of developing attention and awareness. The effects of such meditative trainings often reach beyond mental sharpening: improvements in attention are found together with better emotional balance, greater self-acceptance, reduced stress, and increased feelings of well-being in life.[2] Mindfulness—a specific shift in perception that can be accessed in meditation as well as in the course of a typical day—is an approach with far-reaching effects. Since ADHD can also have far-reaching effects on cognition, emotions, and general sense of self, mindfulness is increasingly recommended for ADHD.[3]

Let's look more closely at what mindfulness is—and what is not.

Being on Automatic Pilot

John is rushing to make an early morning doctor's appointment. Work has been busy and stressful, but he is due for a physical exam. "I hope it doesn't take too long," John thinks as he gets in the car and heads onto the highway. The doctor's office is near John's workplace, so he hopes to still be at work by 9 a.m. after his appointment. Traffic isn't too bad, and in fifteen minutes he is walking into his workplace. Just then his wife calls on his cell phone to remind him to ask the doctor about his snoring. John gasps and realizes that he drove to work instead of the doctor's office! "How could I have spaced out so much?" he wonders as he rushes back out to make his appointment. The answer is simple: his mind was elsewhere and his body automatically took him along his usual route to work.

John's experience of "spacing out" is universal. We all experience moments of being unaware or mindless. In fact, most people are frequently not fully aware of what they're doing throughout day and instead function on "automatic pilot."[4] We're on autopilot whenever we become absentminded or preoccupied with our thoughts or actions. It often happens in situations that don't require new learning, such as when we're engaged in routine or repetitive activities, like walking, eating, or driving.

Overall, automatic-pilot mode can be quite helpful, in that it preserves our mental energy. Imagine being hyperaware of the car and all the aspects of your driving every time you got behind the wheel. Every trip would feel like your first driving lesson, and that would be exhausting.

However, the problem with automatic pilot is that it can make our thinking narrow and inflexible, and it leaves us entrenched in our habits. For example, we can automatically put down our keys when we arrive home, and later have no idea where they are. We can approach a work problem in a conventional way and never ask ourselves, "Is there another way I could do this?" Stress and intense emotions can also kick us into automatic-pilot mode and limit the ways we react to a situation. Many ADHD symptoms happen automatically as well; for example, you may be interrupting without knowing you are doing it, agreeing to do something as a knee-jerk reaction, acting impulsively, losing track of time, or overreacting emotionally over and over again.

Living in Autopilot Can Work for Us...

Kathy has been taking piano lessons since age ten. She remembers how challenging it was to first learn a complicated Mozart piece, but now she doesn't have to pay so much attention. Her fingers "simply know where to go."

Or Against Us

Julie took her white car to a repair shop. The shop gave her a silver loaner car, which she drove to work. After work, she went to the parking lot and started looking for her white car. It took her several seconds to remember she had driven the silver loaner.

What Is Mindfulness?

Alice has been taking a mindfulness class for several weeks. At dinner with her friends, one of them asks, "So, what is mindfulness, really?" Alice explains that mindfulness is paying attention to the present moment. "Like right now," she says, "noticing that we are sitting at a table and talking to each other."

"Of course, on some level we know that we're sitting and talking," Alice continues, "but our attention and awareness are often on what we're saying or planning to say in response to others. Or we're caught up in thinking about the past or the future. Typically, we aren't fully present, fully noticing what it's like to be here together right now. Most of the time we don't have that kind of awareness, unless we actively bring our attention to it."

In contrast to automatic pilot, *mindfulness (or mindful awareness) is a mental state of consistent and flexible attention to the present moment.* Mindfulness also involves a *nonjudgmental attitude:* a way of seeing what is happening around you or inside you *with curiosity, openness, and acceptance.*[5] This kind of perception can lead to enhanced insight, choice, and thoughtful action. In addition, mindfulness can also mean a personal characteristic: so-called trait or dispositional mindfulness. The mindfulness trait is associated with five main facets:[6]

1. *Being nonreactive*   Not automatically reacting to (that is, pushing away or hanging on to) your thoughts or feelings; instead, being able to see them calmly and with some distance.

2. *Observing with awareness*   Paying attention to or spontaneously noticing things such as sensations (for example, the wind on your face); qualities of things you see (colors and shapes); or observing how your thoughts, feelings, and actions interact with each other.

3. *Acting with awareness*   Paying full attention to what you're doing; acknowledging what you're doing as you're doing it; not being absentminded or acting automatically.

4. *Describing with awareness*   Finding words to describe or label what you're thinking, feeling, or experiencing.

5. *Being nonjudgmental toward experience*   Not criticizing yourself for what you think or feel; being open to noticing what's going on inside of you without negative judgment.

In this book I focus on mindfulness as a state of mind that we can enter and exit at any time in the midst of our daily activities, including during ADHD moments. In this approach, mindfulness is more about working with one's attention and attitude in the midst of everyday life than it is about establishing a sitting meditation practice. Formal meditation exercises are important—we will use them here as well—but I've found that including brief and informal mindfulness breaks in the course of daily life is an approach that works very well for ADHD patients.

Spontaneous versus Trained Mindfulness

In everyday language, the word *mindful* often means "remembering to be aware or attentive"; for example, we are mindful (or extra-attentive and aware) of our footsteps when carefully crossing a stream on slippery rocks. Most of us, whether or not we have ADHD, can adopt this mental state for at least a short period of time, so *all of us already have some inherent ability to be mindful.*

The mindfulness state can happen spontaneously or at will. For example, when a beautiful flower catches our attention, or perhaps a child's expression, we often spontaneously become more "present." When we step outside and take in the freshness of the morning, our senses open up and we can feel the moment with more clarity. Through these occasional incidents of spontaneous mindfulness we often sense a deeper connection to ourselves and to the outside world. We also tend to remember the moment more fully.

While mindfulness can happen spontaneously, it is difficult to keep it going consistently in our life. Often our attention is focused on the past or the future—remembering, re-thinking or planning—and the present moment is missed. Furthermore, even if we attend to something in the present, we often do it with a biased attitude or an agenda of some kind: "I know this is going to be like this," or "I want to make this like that." To receive the present-moment experience fully and openly is thus a process of returning to a very basic, unbiased way of perceiving—an ability that is strengthened by a dedicated mindfulness practice.

There are many different programs that offer mindfulness training. Such programs range from mindfulness meditation groups at local meditation centers to mindfulness-training classes at universities and health clinics. In clinical, secular settings, mindfulness is often taught in the form of Mindfulness-Based Stress Reduction (MBSR)—a pioneering, eight-week course developed by Jon Kabat-Zinn at the University of Massachusetts.[7] MBSR is also the model or basis for new programs that tailor mindfulness training to specific problems such as depression and anxiety (Mindfulness-Based Cognitive Therapy, or MBCT[8]) and ADHD (such as our Mindful Awareness Practices for ADHD). Other therapies that use mindfulness exercises include Dialectical Behavioral Therapy (DBT), Acceptance Commitment Therapy (ACT), and Gestalt therapy.[9]

Turning On the Mindful State of Mind

As I've explained, mindfulness is something that we can actually turn on or off throughout our day, as we go about our usual activities. The main question then becomes: how do we shift out of autopilot and into mindfulness?

The answer lies in adjusting the two key components of mindfulness: attention and attitude. We bring our attention to the present moment and take on an attitude of openness and curiosity.

THE TWO KEY ASPECTS OF MINDFULNESS

1. Attention to the present moment
2. An attitude of openness and curiosity

Let's explore the two key aspects of mindfulness with the following exercise.

- Look around and find something that catches your eye.
- Bring close attention to it and make it the object of your full focus. See if you can detect your attitude toward the object. Do you like it or dislike it? Do you sense yourself as nonjudgmental, or do you feel yourself wanting to compare, analyze, or criticize it?
- If you don't like it, see if for a moment you can increase a feeling of dislike or rejection of the object. Notice how you are when you do that.
- Now see if you can shift to a stance of openness and

curiosity toward the object. Be nonjudgmental and notice how that feels to you.

- Next, look around, noticing things around you with full attention and openness and curiosity. It may help to imagine that you just came from another planet and are looking at the things around you for the first time.
- Consciously note the fact that *you're paying attention right now in this specific way*.
- Can you feel a sense of enhanced awareness? Note whatever your experience is in this moment. There is no right or wrong way of doing this, as long as you notice your experience with enhanced awareness—even if what you find is that it is hard for you to do an aspect of this exercise.

This specific way of paying attention can be applied to things in the outside world as well as to what is happening inside of you. For example, you can bring mindful awareness to the flavor of your coffee while sipping it at work. This can deepen your moment of relaxation and make you less frantic and more focused afterward. Or you can be mindfully aware of your mind, body, and behavior as you speak with your boss. For instance, maybe your mind is distracted, maybe you feel tension in your neck, or maybe you tend to interrupt. Mindfulness can help you notice attention shifts, thoughts, feelings, body sensations, and impulses with new clarity. Such enhanced awareness can later help you recognize when ADHD shows up in your life, and help you relate to it—as well as work through it—with compassion and skill.

Q: I've heard about Transcendental Meditation (TM). What is the difference between TM and mindfulness?

Attention is at the heart of all meditation practices and we can divide different meditation styles into two basic categories: (1) focused attention, or concentration training, and (2) open, or receptive, attention training.

The Hindu practice of TM is an example of concentration practice. In this meditation, attention is typically focused on a single point, such as a word (mantra), or breathing. Such repeated attention to a single point trains concentration and can lead to a state of absorption or a feeling of an altered state.

Mindfulness meditation (also known as Vipassana in the Buddhist context) is an example of open attention practice. While it includes some focused attention practices (for example, mindfulness of the breath), mindfulness emphasizes training in being alert and receptive to whatever happens from moment to moment.

Meditation teachers often see synergy between focused and open attention training. A helpful analogy of a wooden stick says that focused attention (TM) and open awareness (mindfulness) trainings are like the ends of the same wooden stick: If you pick up one end, the other will follow. Research studies confirm this overlap in meditation techniques and show that mindfulness practice can train diverse aspects of attention including focused attention[10] and that TM practice can increase the ability for mindfulness.[11]

See the table below for some examples of concentration and open attention meditation exercises.

	ATTENTION SPECTRUM Focused ——————————————— Open	
Placement of attention	Examples of Meditation Practices	
Outside of yourself	Focusing on a candle's light	Noticing incoming sounds "Taking-in the surroundings through your senses" while in nature Paying attention to space, absence, or timelessness around you

	ATTENTION SPECTRUM	
	Focused ————————————————— Open	
Placement of attention	Examples of Meditation Practices	
Inside of yourself	Focusing on counting breaths	Noticing the changing flow of thoughts
	Focusing on repeating one word (e.g., a mantra in TM)	

A hallmark of mindfulness is that experiences are monitored with awareness; this is how we avoid falling into full absorption or getting lost in the experience. Of course in practice there may be moments of feeling lost in thinking or doing. However, mindfulness practice encourages returning to the present moment so that, if necessary, the attention can be pulled back, refocused, or in some way readjusted so the mind is neither overly engrossed nor too scattered. This dual nature of mindfulness—focus and monitoring of attention—makes it an antidote to hyperfocus as well as inattention. Over time, mindfulness practice develops not only awareness but also *discernment* of what things are helpful to focus on and when.

It's important to note that mindfulness is also a practice of being alert and attentive yet relaxed. This is in contrast to how we tend to pay attention in daily life: with effort, tension, and stress. Mindfulness involves watching your experience and allowing it to reveal itself to you. It's less about making an effort and more about allowing yourself to open to the present moment. For that reason we often say mindfulness is "dropping into" awareness. Keep that in mind as we go through the eight steps in part 2 of this book. I will often ask you to do mindful practices that at first may seem like a lot of effort. However, the practices are truly an invitation *to let go* of doing things in an old way and *allow* the present moment to come to you. All you have to do is watch, know, and discern.

Mindfulness and ADHD: Polar Opposites?

At first glance, ADHD and mindfulness would seem to be diametrically opposed: ADHD is characterized by moments of distraction and spacing out; mindfulness is characterized by moments of full attention and presence. At first glance this contrast is obvious, but that's not the whole story. In my clinical work with adults with ADHD, I have found that many of these adults, once they experience mindful awareness, seem "natural" in their capacity for a curious attitude. Their ability for openness to new experiences is quite apparent, and they can also be quite creative in how they approach and practice mindfulness.

A research study done by the ADHD researcher Susan Smalley at UCLA supports my clinical observation and suggests that while the attention aspect of mindfulness is often difficult for adults with ADHD, the other aspects of mindfulness may in fact be easier for adults with ADHD than it is for others.[12] Self-transcendence (the ability to step outside of oneself) is positively correlated with having ADHD and being mindful. So while mindfulness training will challenge you to train your attention, it can, and mostly likely will, tap into your other natural strengths. In the next chapter we will further explore the ways that ADHD and mindfulness intersect.

Q: Isn't "being in a moment" what causes problems for people with ADHD?

It's true that if you have ADHD it's easy to get lost in what you're doing or to attend to the "wrong thing," depending on what grabs your attention from moment to moment. This bouncing around of your attention often happens automatically or impulsively, and you can spend much time doing something different than what you first set out to do.

Mindfulness is a practice of awareness and remembering. You not only bring your awareness to the present moment, but you learn to pay attention to where your attention is going. When you notice your attention wandering from the task at hand, you bring your attention back to the intended task, again and again. This monitoring and remembering is called meta-awareness, and it helps you stay connected to your goals and resist distractions and diversions. Even if you get lost in the moment, with mindfulness you realize it sooner and can self-correct.

A Taste of Mindfulness Practice

Next time you have tea or coffee, notice the aroma, the warmth, and the taste with full attention. Notice how this experience is different from your usual way of drinking it. Brief mindfulness practice can be as simple as that.

2   Mindfulness and Self-Regulation in ADHD

In a famous study done in the late 1960s at Stanford University, Dr. Walter Mischel (a psychologist specializing in the theory of human personality) asked a group of four-year-olds to each sit at a table in a room, alone. On the table in front of each child was a plate with a marshmallow on it. The children were told that if they could wait for fifteen minutes without eating the marshmallow, they would get another one as a reward.[1] Well, waiting fifteen minutes to eat a yummy marshmallow — placed right within the child's reach — is a test of true willpower for a four-year-old. I encourage you to check out the reenactment videos (do an Internet search using "YouTube marshmallow test") and see how different children deal with the task. Some squirm in their seat, some distract themselves, some physically restrain their hands by sitting on them, and some simply give up. It's fascinating to watch their attempts to practice delayed gratification.

In the original study, the researchers followed the group of children into adulthood and found that those who had been able to delay gratification on the marshmallow test at age four generally did better in life. Compared to the kids who ate the marshmallow right away, those who could wait did better on collage entrance tests, had better career and relationship trajectories, and were less moody, less envious, and more cooperative.[2] In short, they had greater capacity for *self-regulation*.

Self-regulation is similar to self-control and includes self-monitoring and self-correction; it is our conscious ability to direct our attention, thoughts, emotions, impulses, and actions. Self-regulation also includes self-talk and other strategies that help us to delay immediate gratification in pursuit of a future goal. We begin to develop basic self-regulation skills in childhood, and the process never ends. However, for adults with ADHD, altered brain function and cognitive deficits may create lifelong problems with these skills. Symptoms such as being impulsive, moody, impatient, or easily distracted are all common in ADHD. These behaviors often translate into difficulties at work, at school, and with relationships. Indeed, these problems can, and often do, prevent people from achieving their goals. At the very least, problems with self-regulation can lead to much frustration, stress, and self-doubt. Dr. Russell Barkley, a prominent psychologist and an expert in the ADHD field, in fact calls ADHD "the disorder of self-regulation."[3]

In explaining ADHD, Dr. Barkley also applies the concept of *self-regulation strength*.[4] This concept, related to willpower, says that self-regulation strength is a limited resource—a tank or a pool—that can be depleted by using it.[5] This is true for everyone, but in ADHD, the self-regulation tank may be smaller to begin with and may run out faster with difficult tasks. Once the self-regulation tank is depleted, it is easier to have "failures of self-regulation," for example having an emotional meltdown or overeating after a mentally taxing task. Strategies that relax and replenish can restore one's reservoir of willpower and are thus helpful in ADHD. These strategies include: times of relaxation such as meditation, positive emotions, self-talk that is encouraging, time of play, physical exercise, adequate breaks, or even having a snack that increases blood glucose. Motivational strategies such imagery, or physical reminders of or talking about future rewards can also help.

The good news is that with understanding and the right treatment, you can learn to manage your ADHD and the self-regulation difficulties that come with it. On your ADHD journey—yes, it is a journey—mindfulness can be of tremendous help, as it teaches effective self-regulation strategies and can help replenish the self-regulation tank. With these strategies, you can enhance your well-being, build resilience, and not just live but thrive with ADHD.

What Is Self-Regulation, Exactly?

Self-regulation isn't a word we often use in daily life, yet it describes something we do many times each day. It's also an important concept in understanding ADHD and mindfulness. So let's look at this concept more closely.

By not acting on the feeling of impatience when standing in a checkout line, you're practicing conscious self-regulation to achieve a goal (paying for your groceries so you can leave the store). If you're a parent, you're probably challenged to consciously self-regulate more than you ever had to before—as when you come home from a long day at work and your child wants attention, and you stop yourself from showing your annoyance and tiredness.

There are many ways in which we may attempt to self-regulate—some successful and some not. The following is an example with many instances of different self-regulation strategies.

Mary's Story

Mary woke up one morning thinking about her long-overdue work report. Immediately, she had a sinking sensation in her stomach and felt overwhelmed. The report had been hanging over her head for a while, and she'd been trying to ignore or push down her feelings of discomfort while distracting herself with other tasks.

This morning, however, she allowed herself to experience the unpleasant feelings more fully, just for a moment. As she did this, she became aware of how afraid she was of the effort that would be required to write the report, as well as her anticipated failure. As she faced the fear, however, she developed some distance from it. She decided to motivate herself for the task. She thought to herself, "By 9 a.m. I'm going to be at the computer and work on it for a couple of hours and then take a break. It's going to be hard, but I know I can do it!" She immediately felt better, and the overwhelmed feeling was gone. She set the alarm to remind her when to start working.

As 9 a.m. rolled around and the alarm reminder prompted her, Mary sat down at the computer. First she started browsing some news websites. She was procrastinating. Thirty minutes passed, and she was still exploring the latest events. Her favorite topic, women's soccer, was at the forefront of the news, and she loved browsing through different stories. She finally noticed the time and felt a moment of indecision. "Do I go back to work or do I continue reading?" she asked herself. She really wanted to keep reading and felt irritated that she had work to do. Yet she pulled herself back and closed the news sites. She put her attention back on her work and started writing. Periodically she had an urge to check and see what was happening in the media, but she resisted these urges and kept working without interruption for about an hour.

However, as she wrote her mind started wandering off—a lot. She also felt like she was repeating herself in her writing, and her thoughts were disorganized. Since Mary has ADHD and dyslexia, writing is often a challenge, and she finds herself either hyperfocused on a single paragraph or, alternately, overwhelmed with the entire task. She started feeling bad about herself and utterly discouraged. "I'm just not a good writer!" she thought. "This is useless! I'm going to fail! I hate this!" She got up from her computer, went to the kitchen, and grabbed a chocolate bar to munch on. The food distracted her and provided some positive feeling, but she was still feeling bad inside. She decided to call a friend.

As she spoke to her friend, Mary talked about her struggle with writing and how awful she felt about the whole process. Her friend sympathized with the difficulty but also encouraged her to persist. "Why don't you write an outline first?" the friend suggested. "Then write on each section for about thirty minutes every day." These suggestions gave Mary a new faith in herself and a new perspective. She again sat down at her desk and finally came up with an outline. She wrote her first paragraph, too, then decided to do other things for the rest of the day. She felt that thirty minutes a day was doable for her, and she decided that she could plan to work on small sections over the next several days.

In this story, Mary used several approaches to self-regulation.

COMMON SELF-REGULATION STRATEGIES
- Ignoring, suppressing, or pushing down an uncomfortable thought or feeling
- Facing the unpleasant feeling
- Self-talk for guidance or motivation
- Using reminders or alarms
- Inhibiting a response
- Removing the distraction
- Getting away physically from a situation
- Eating to feel better

Although successful self-regulation sometimes requires staying with the unpleasant situation, at other times it helps to move away from it. In Mary's case, she needed to face her underlying fears of failure in order to stop procrastinating. However, later on, she needed to step away from the work to regain a balanced perspective.

Take a moment and reflect on the following questions: What self-regulation strategies have you used? What works for you? Which ones don't work?

Self-Regulation and Executive Functions

The difficulty in self-regulating with ADHD is related to a weakness in *executive functions* (frequently abbreviated as EF).[6] EF is a catch-all term for a number of skills that have to do with directing our thinking, feelings, and actions and achieving goals.

Examples of Executive Functions

Impulse control: The ability to withhold a response or action (to allow for reflection and assessment)

Working memory: The ability to keep verbal or nonverbal information in mind while doing a task; a kind of internal "clipboard"

Emotional control: The ability to modulate intense emotions, to calm oneself

Self-monitoring: The ability to "check in" on one's thoughts, feelings, and actions—and if needed, self-correct

Task management: The ability to initiate, persist with, and complete a task; also includes the ability to shift flexibly from one task or situation to another

Planning, prioritizing, and organizing: The ability to plan tasks over time, break complex tasks down, and keep spaces, things, or ideas organized

Time management: The ability to be realistic about how long things take; demonstrating timeliness; having a good sense of time

Commonly, executive functions are compared to the skills of effective leaders, such as those of a corporate executive or an orchestra director. For example, the executive has to remember the overall company goals and make decisions that meet the goals without getting distracted by other agendas. But with EF, we are leading ourselves in our daily lives. You could say that executive functions are self-leadership skills.

Dr. Barkley's work shows that most adults with ADHD report difficulties with tasks that require EFs, so if you have ADHD, this may be the case for you too.[7] For example, you can have many ideas but likely have trouble focusing and prioritizing, since you may think everything is equally important. You may feel paralyzed, not knowing where to begin, or you may sometimes impulsively start several projects at once. You may have trouble initiating a task, staying on task, or transitioning out of a task. You may also have trouble estimating how much time you have, and so you end up always trying to squeeze too many last-minute tasks in before you leave your house. It may be hard to keep an intention in mind, inhibit an impulse, think flexibly, or shift from one thing to another. At times your brain may function like a slow computer getting in the way of a timely response.

Treating Self-Regulation Difficulties in ADHD

The self-regulation difficulties in ADHD are often addressed with stimulant medications, such as Ritalin and Adderall, the mainstay of ADHD treatment. Medications can be tremendously helpful for some adults with ADHD. Both stimulant and nonstimulant medications are available, and for many adults these treatments can help overcome their ADHD symptoms.

However, medications are not always the solution: side effects or coexisting medical conditions can limit their use. Others with ADHD prefer to learn skills that help them minimize lifelong reliance on medications or help with the symptoms that remain, despite medications. Many people do best using a combination of medications and other nondrug approaches. As a result, today there is a growing interest among ADHD adults and their doctors to try nonpharmaceutical treatments that build intrinsic self-awareness and self-regulation skills.

Promising new tools for treating ADHD include:

- Computer-based programs to improve cognition (for example, working memory)
- Diverse programs used in educational therapy
- Neurofeedback training (also called brainwave biofeedback)
- Cognitive-behavioral therapy and other psychotherapies
- Coaching
- Mind-body exercises (such as yoga or meditation)

- Physical exercise
- Exposure to nature ("green therapy")
- Nutrition and supplements (such as fish oil)

Most of the drug-free approaches to ADHD require further study to confirm their usefulness. For mindfulness and related mind-body approaches specifically, the research field is still young but growing and showing increasing promise. This research currently includes several studies with children and adults with ADHD.[8] As mentioned earlier, our pilot study at UCLA trained mindfulness in a group of teens and adults with ADHD, and in 2010 the program was adapted with good results for elementary children by Anna Uliando at Deakin University in Melbourne, Australia. Studies done in Germany showed that an approach derived from dialectical behavioral therapy—which has mindfulness as one of its key components—improves symptoms in ADHD adults.[9] Participants in these studies rated mindfulness as one of the most helpful parts of the program.[10]

In a pilot mindfulness study conducted by Dr. Nirbhay Singh at ONE Research Institute in Virginia, two mothers, each with an ADHD child, received mindfulness training in order to see the effect of parental mindfulness on the child's behavior. Afterward, the mothers reported enhanced compliance in their children, even though no specific parenting instructions were given to the mothers. Moreover, the effect was even greater when the children themselves were given similar mindfulness training.[11]

Dr. Saskia van der Oord and her colleagues at the University of Amsterdam conducted a study of eight-week group mindfulness trainings for twenty-two children aged eight to twelve, all with ADHD.[12] Parents (mostly mothers and one father) of these children completed a parallel mindful parenting program. The effect of the training was measured by having parents and children's teachers fill out questionnaires before, immediately after, and eight weeks after the training. Overall, the parents reported improvements in their children's ADHD symptoms (but not ODD symptoms) as well as improvments in their own ADHD symptoms, overactive parenting, and parental stress.

The study did not, however, find significant changes in teacher-rated ADHD symptoms in the children.

In addition to mindfulness techniques, other mind-body modalities are being researched as treatments for ADHD. These include pilot studies of yoga for eight-to-twelve-year-old children with ADHD and their parents,[13] Transcendental Meditation with eleven-to-fourteen-year-old students with ADHD,[14] and tai chi for adolescents (ages twelve to eighteen) with ADHD.[15] Most of the up-to-date studies in mind-body treatment for ADHD have been small and without a control group; however, their overall promising results, inexpensive treatments, and minimal—if any—side effects call for more research like this in ADHD.

What We Know about Mindfulness—and the Implications for ADHD

In this section we'll review the benefits of mindfulness practice, including enhanced attention control, memory, emotional regulation, coping with stress, and relationships with others—all of which can be areas of challenge for adults living with ADHD.

In this discussion, I describe several notable mindfulness studies done in the general population (research that was not focused on individuals with ADHD). Keep in mind that confirming research specifically with ADHD participants is yet to be done. Here I hope to engender your curiosity and excitement about the growing science of mindfulness and show you how mindfulness intersects with the many aspects of ADHD.

Attention Control

Because of its name, ADHD is often perceived as a deficit in attention, but more accurately, *it's a deficit in attention regulation.* In other words, ADHD makes it more difficult to have appropriate attention at the right time. In different contexts, a lack of focus or hyperfocus can be a problem for the same person with

ADHD. Difficulties with transitions in focus, such as disengaging from a task and starting a new one, are also common.

HOW CAN MINDFULNESS HELP?

Through mindfulness practice, you become more frequently aware of your attention and able to direct it at will. For example, in this book's eight-step program, you'll do an exercise of focusing on the breath. While doing so, you notice when you're focused on the breath, and when you're distracted, and you practice redirecting your attention back to the breath. This strengthens the ability to concentrate. In later exercises, you'll also learn how to open the field of your attention and notice whatever arises from moment to moment—a practice often called "open monitoring." This trains us in alert, flexible, and receptive attention. Such attention is thought to promote self-reflection and insight.

WHAT THE RESEARCH SHOWS
Mindfulness and Attention Control

Increasing numbers of studies are looking at the effects of mindfulness on attention. For example, research by Dr. Amishi Jha done at the University of Pennsylvania showed that adults who participated in either an eight-week mindfulness class or one-month meditation retreat showed improvements in different aspects of attention as compared to control group. The kind of improvements depended on the type of training and prior experience with meditation.[16]

An interesting collaboration between Dr. Katherine MacLean at Johns Hopkins University, researchers at University of California–Davis, and the meditation teacher and scholar Alan Wallace studied a group of adults in an intensive three-month meditation training. The training involved up to five hours a day of meditation, including sustained attention on the breath. After the three months of practice, the participants had sharpened visual perception and were more alert when paying attention—changes that may facilitate the ability for prolonged sustained attention.[17]

Finally, a 2010 review of twenty-three controlled mindfulness studies that included attention measures concluded that early phases of mindfulness training are associated with significant improvement in selective and executive attention whereas later phases (that is, the "open monitoring practice") bring improvement in alert, sustained attention.[18] The review calls for larger studies, but it nonetheless confirms the potential of mindfulness to improve attention.

Memory

Adults with ADHD often complain of memory problems. For example, they can complain of having trouble remembering a phone number they just looked up or having to constantly look at the recipe when cooking something. These short-term memory difficulties are related to working memory, a component of executive function.

In daily life, working memory functions as an internal "clipboard" that helps us hold information in mind as we perform complex tasks. The information we retain can be nonverbal—such as pictures and memories—or it can be verbal—for instance, something we have read, something someone told us, or internal self-talk. In ADHD both kinds of working memory are weaker, and the deficit makes it hard to learn, remember, and follow inner knowledge and rules.

HOW CAN MINDFULNESS HELP?

Just like attention, working memory is intimately involved in mindfulness practice. In all mindfulness exercises you have a set intention for the practice period (such as, "I am going to notice the breath"), and you must frequently remember the intention. If your mind wanders off, part of the practice is to remind yourself what you are supposed to be doing and return to it. Similarly, in daily life, mindfulness calls for frequently "remembering to be present." In this way, working memory is continuously engaged in mindfulness practice and is "exercised."

In addition to working memory mindfulness practice is often thought to also enhance memory for events by expanding the breadth and depth of the information that is observed. Mindfulness calls for full attention, full "taking-in" of an experience, which can help us recall the experience later on. (The exercise "Tuning In to the Five Senses" in Step 1 of the program demonstrates this quality of mindfulness.)

📖 WHAT THE RESEARCH SHOWS
Mindfulness and Memory

So far, science has given us only few studies on the effects of mindfulness on memory, but the research done so far suggests a positive effect on working memory. For example, significant improvements in working memory were found in a group of adults attending a mindfulness retreat.[19] Another study, headed by Dr. Amishi Jha, found that soldiers under training stress who participated in a mindfulness class preserved their working memory, while soldiers who did not receive such training experienced depletion of their working memory.[20] In a UCLA study that looked at executive function skills (including working memory) in second- and third-grade children receiving mindfulness training in their school, the results showed that children starting out with poor executive functions had significant gains in EF after receiving the eight-week mindfulness training.[21]

Emotion Regulation

Emotional regulation means the ability to balance or modulate one's emotions. It means not blowing up when you're angry, but it also means not suppressing anger so much that you never speak up when something is wrong. Good emotional regulation leads to psychological resilience and being able to control strong impulses. We know that this skill is often impaired in ADHD. Studies have shown adults with ADHD have more difficulty controlling impulsive reactions than their non-ADHD peers and that these difficulties can lead to problems at work and in relationships.[22] Adults with ADHD are also more prone to depression, anxiety, and substance abuse—conditions that are often fueled by underlying problems with emotion regulation.

HOW CAN MINDFULNESS HELP?

Mindfulness can help you become more aware of your feelings and help you deal with them in a compassionate and balanced way. In mindfulness practice, you learn to watch your feelings from a "witnessing" perspective, without pushing them away or getting flooded by them. You also practice labeling your feelings (that is, putting words on the experience) in a nonjudgmental way. Such strategies help you to step back from strong emotional reactions and resist impulsive actions. (Step 6 of the eight-step program presents several mindful strategies for transforming difficult emotions.)

WHAT THE RESEARCH SHOWS

Mindfulness and Emotion Regulation

There is good research indicating that mindfulness helps with emotional regulation.[23] The best studies come from the study of depression, where MBCT (Mindfulness-Based Cognitive Therapy) has been shown to be effective in preventing relapse into depression.[24] One well-designed study by Dr. Willem Kuyken at University of Exeter showed that including MBCT in maintenance treatment for depression not only helped patients decrease their relapse risk but also allowed the majority of them to get off their antidepressant medications.[25]

The effects of mindfulness on emotions have also been studied from a different angle: looking at the capacity for mindfulness as a personality trait (so-called dispositional mindfulness) and seeing how it relates to overall psychological well-being. Drs. Kirk Brown and Richard Ryan at University of Rochester have shown that those high in dispositional mindfulness had overall decreased levels of anxiety and depression, and they were less prone to neuroticism, rumination, and low self-esteem. They also tended to have higher emotional intelligence and positive emotions.[26]

When it comes to impulsive emotions such anger or craving, mindfulness-based therapies have also been promising. For example, a pilot study conducted by Dr. Singh (mentioned above) has shown that a mindfulness meditation in which attention is shifted from an anger-producing situation to sensations at the soles of the feet had the effect of decreasing verbal and physical aggression in three psychiatric patients who had frequently been hospitalized as a result of their anger management problems.[27] Other studies have also shown that impulses such as craving in addictions and binge eating can be ameliorated with mindfulness training.[28]

Coping with Stress

Having ADHD can be stressful, and the stress often starts early in life. The quality of life for children with ADHD has been shown to be lower not only compared to healthy children but even in comparison to children with chronic asthma.[29] ADHD children often report feeling different and socially isolated, and many struggle with academic difficulties.

Adults with ADHD commonly continue to experience stress in college, in work situations, or in their relationships. Unfortunately, financial difficulties, substance abuse, driving accidents, and divorce are more likely to occur in the lives of adults with ADHD.[30] In my own practice, I see many ADHD adults who are stressed and overwhelmed. They frequently feel behind and are constantly trying to catch up on what they need to do. They often describe themselves as "running on empty." They may be living with ADHD, but they are not thriving with ADHD.

Like other mind-body techniques, mindfulness practice can help your body relax—which counteracts the physiological effects of intense or chronic stress. Setting aside time for mindfulness, even for just few minutes at a time (for instance, taking time to notice your breath many times during the course of the day), can make a big difference in how much the daily stress affects you. The practice also leads to increased experience of positive emotions such as joy and well-being.

Mindfulness also promotes a positive shift in how we relate to all of our experiences. For example, during a stressful situation, mindfulness encourages curiosity and compassion instead of shame, despair, or frustration. How you see things, how you relate to the circumstances of your life, makes a big difference in your stress level.

📖   WHAT THE RESEARCH SHOWS

Mindfulness and Stress

One of first ways mindfulness was introduced to the medical world was for the treatment of chronic pain and stress using a pioneering program called the Mindfulness-Based Stress Reduction program (MBSR) that was developed by Dr. Jon Kabat-Zinn at the University of Massachusetts in the 1970s. Since then many studies—of people ranging from cancer patients to medical students to parents—have shown that MBSR can reduce stress regardless of its cause.[31] The reduction in stress is often reported to be accompanied by increased feelings of positive emotions, vitality, and self-acceptance.

MBSR training has also been shown to improve body and brain functioning. For example, a study by Dr. Richard Davidson at the University of Wisconsin took a group of biotech employees and gave half of the group mindfulness training for eight weeks. Everyone in the group also got a flu vaccine at the beginning of the study, and all of the participants also had their brain waves measured via electroencephalograph before and after the eight-week period. Compared to those who did not get the mindfulness training, participants who received the training had a better response to the vaccine and showed a shift in their brain waves consistent with becoming more optimistic.[32]

Relationships

ADHD often comes with increased struggles in relationships. Families with ADHD children often have increased family stress, conflict, poorer adjustment to married life, and depression, and adults with ADHD have high rates of marital conflict and a higher divorce rate than their non-ADHD peers.[33] But the negative effects on relationships are not just with others; they also extend to the relationship the ADHD person has with himself or herself. Low self-esteem and self-doubt are common in ADHD.[34]

HOW CAN MINDFULNESS HELP?

Mindfulness teaches how to manage negative emotions and communicate thoughtfully with others. Therefore, it tends to increase satisfaction in relationships, help with parenting, and refine one's social skills.

In addition, mindfulness promotes a more compassionate and intimate relationship with oneself. Dr. Dan Siegel, a psychiatrist and an expert on the role of early attachment in mental health, has aptly described mindfulness as a practice of attunement to yourself—a means of fostering a nurturing, attentive relationship with yourself.[35] Such close attunement is often compromised in a child's early years, and this can create a lifelong barrier in knowing yourself. Mindfulness practice helps overcome that barrier, and this in turn can increase the capacity for intimacy with others.

📖 WHAT THE RESEARCH SHOWS

Mindfulness and Relationships

In the scientific literature, mindfulness has been proposed as means of improving relationships; however the number of relevant studies is still small. As mentioned earlier in the chapter, Dr. Singh's research suggested that mindfulness training for mothers had a positive effect on their children with ADHD. One study focusing on romantic relationships showed that mindfulness-based intervention for couples decreased relationship stress, increased relationship satisfaction, and improved a couple's experience of relating, feeling closeness, and being accepting of one another.[36]

Another study explored the effects of meditation on the interaction between a therapist and his or her patient. The study compared a group of psychotherapists in training who meditated right before seeing their patients to a group of similar psychotherapists, who also meditated but at a time that was not so close to their meeting with patients. The study showed that *the patients* of therapists who meditated right before their sessions had more improvement in their symptoms and reported more satisfaction with the treatment than the patients of therapists who did not meditate before sessions.[37]

Training the Brain: The Power of Neuroplasticity

In the last several years there has been a lot of excitement about the discovery that the brain can grow and change throughout life—a quality called *neuroplasticity*. This term is derived from two words: *neuro*, or related to the brain, and *plastic*, which means pliable or changeable. The brain has been shown to change in response to one's experiences, especially when the experience is repeated. Brain scientists used to think that neuroplasticity was a feature of the brain only during childhood, but now we know that the brain actively adapts throughout one's life.[38] This discovery has fueled much interest in different brain-training technologies.

Examples of Neuroplasticity

- Taxi drivers have to keep much visual and spatial information in their minds as they memorize directions and maps. A British neuroimaging study comparing the brains of taxi drivers with those of non–taxi drivers showed that the hippocampus—the part of the brain that is important for memory—was thicker or more developed in taxi drivers.[39]
- Children with ADHD who played computer games designed to enhance working memory had enhanced brain activation in the prefrontal cortex after five weeks of training.[40]

Attention is a key factor in neuroplasticity. Where we direct our attention determines which neural circuits become engaged and modified. This was nicely demonstrated in a study in which two groups of monkeys were exposed to the same environment —sounds and finger taps—however, one group was trained to pay attention to a sound frequency while another group was trained to pay attention to frequency of the finger taps. Later on, the groups were compared on how their brain function changed. The startling finding was that the monkeys who paid attention to the sound frequency had more-developed auditory cortexes while the other group showed no changes in that region. Thus, despite similar environments—and overall similar experiences—the monkey's purposeful placement of attention shaped where in the brain neural changes occurred.[41]

Meditation as a Way to Stimulate Healthy Neuroplasticity

Understanding neuroplasticity has revolutionized our thinking about meditation. We realized that by repeatedly engaging our brains in a positive way through meditation, we can potentially affect the function and even the structure of our brains.

Research studies with long-term meditators are supporting this notion. For example, Dr. Sarah Lazar at Harvard University showed that long-term meditators had thicker (or more developed) brain regions related to attention, self-monitoring, and emotional processing when compared to an average person. Also, the prefrontal cortex of meditators appeared to resist the typical age-related thinning.[42] Another study, by Dr. Heleen Slagter at the University of Amsterdam in the Netherlands, looked at so-called attention blink — a finding that when two pieces of information are presented quickly, one after another, the brain does not perceive the second piece of information because it is still processing the first piece. In this study, long-term meditators were more apt to perceive both pieces of information than were a control group of nonmeditators. Overall, this study suggested that long-term meditators' brains were more efficient in how they processed incoming information.[43]

How much do you have to practice meditation to affect the brain in a meaningful way? This question continues to be explored. It is likely that changing brain structure with mindfulness requires at least several weeks, if not months, of consistent practice. Just like with physical exercise, you may feel good after only one workout, but developing stamina and increasing your fitness will take several weeks of training — and changing your muscle structure will take even longer. And as with physical exercise, the more meditation you do, with more intensity, the greater the effect.

A couple of studies do suggest that you may not have to devote yourself to years of mindfulness meditation practice before seeing some positive changes in the brain. A study done through a collaboration between Dr. Yi-Yuan Tang from Dalian University of Technology in China and researchers at the University of

Oregon suggested improvements in attention after five days of meditation training.[44] A study at Massachusetts General Hospital led by Dr. Britta Hölzel showed increases in gray matter after an eight-week MBSR course.[45] In the latter study, the affected regions were those known to play a role in learning and memory, processing emotions, thinking about self, and ability to take diverse perspectives.

For our purposes, it is important to note that neuroimaging studies of mindfulness show that mindfulness practice appears to enhance the function of the very brain regions that are also affected in ADHD, namely the prefrontal cortex and the anterior cingulate cortex. These brain regions are critical for self-regulation: control of attention, thinking, and emotions. Although studies that look at brain changes of ADHD children and adults before and after meditation are not yet available, this is an exciting area ripe for further exploration.

3   Getting Ready for the Eight-Step Program

This chapter gives you an overview and practice tips in preparation to begin the eight-step program for using mindfulness to improve attention and find greater emotional balance. (For further discussion of some questions that commonly come up when doing this program, see "FAQ" at the end of the book.)

Mindfulness Is a Playful Practice

For some of you, just seeing the words "meditation" or "eight-step program" may seem like a daunting project involving a lot of work. If you've had a previous negative experience with meditation, you may especially doubt your own abilities to learn mindfulness. But fear not: mindfulness at its heart is an exploration, a journey that involves as much resting, letting go, and playfulness as it involves planning and effort. It is also *your* journey: make it fit your life and your preferences. For example, while I recommend that you give yourself one to two weeks to try practices described in each step before moving on to the next one, you can always take more or less time, come back to a step when you need to, or take a break between steps.

Formal versus Informal Practices

In the eight-step program you will learn two types of mindfulness practice that complement one another: formal and informal practice.

Formal practice is what we typically think of as traditional meditation practice: setting aside some time to do a silent sitting or walking meditation. An audio CD is provided with this book to guide and support you in this kind of practice. (The audio program is also available as a free download at www.shambhala .com/MindfulnessPrescription.)

Informal practice is being mindfully aware in the midst of your daily activities. It is about bringing attention to the present moment, anytime, anywhere, in the course of your day. One of my patients calls it "mindfulness on the go."

Mental Training Is Like Physical Training

You can think of mindfulness practice as mental training similar to physical exercise. *Formal practice* is like having a regular gym routine or another regular activity (for instance, putting in ten minutes every morning on a treadmill or always taking a mile walk in the evening after supper). *Informal practice* is like looking for opportunities to be active in the course of your day (for example, choosing to take the stairs instead of an elevator when you are at work). Both activities help get you physically fit, especially if you take the stairs many times throughout the day.

Similarly, both types of mindfulness practice are valuable and can reinforce each other. And while many of the practices presented in this book are described as formal practices, you quickly come to realize that the same exercises can also be practiced as informal mindfulness. For example, you can practice the sound-breath-body meditation as a formal ten-minute sitting meditation, or you can bring mindful awareness to your breath, your body movement, and the sounds around you many times throughout your day.

Length: The formal practices in this book range from five to fifteen minutes in length. They can be done with or without the audio program included on the audio CD. Many people find it helpful to begin by following along with the audio program. As you become familiar with the practices, you can experiment, doing them on your own or sitting for longer periods of time. The more you practice, the more adept you will become at bringing mindfulness into your life.

Posture: Formal mindfulness practices are typically done while sitting. You don't have to sit in any exotic or ritualized way. Just assume an upright yet relaxed posture, which will help you stay alert and minimize physical strain. I'll often invite you to sit in a "posture of dignity," in command of your body, but not rigid. Eyes can be closed, or they can be open with the gaze directed downward and resting in one spot.

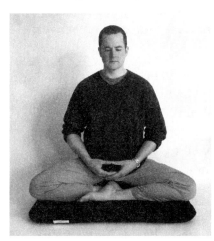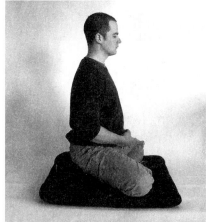

Location: Sitting meditation can be done in a chair with good back support or on the floor in a cross-legged position using a meditation cushion. If you use a cushion, make sure your knees are resting on the floor or mat. Use the cushion as a wedge underneath your buttocks to help your

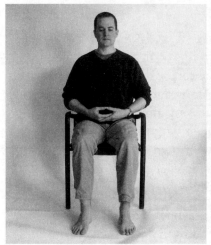 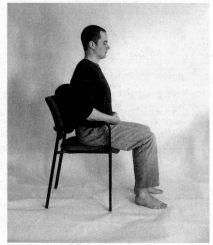

knees reach the floor. If you are not flexible enough for your knees to touch the floor, use a rolled blanket or a pillow under each knee for additional support. Whether sitting in a chair or on a cushion, rest the hands on the lap or below the belly button. Any seat that is easily available to you can work. One of my ADHD patients is a dentist and uses his dental chair to do mindfulness meditation between seeing patients.

Difficulties: If, at any point, sitting still becomes too difficult, as an act of kindness to yourself and your ADHD, feel free to shift your position, do mindful walking instead of sitting (described in more detail in step 1), or simply stop and return to it later. Although the bottom line of this program is to challenge yourself, you should also listen to what is right for you.

Alone or with others? Most people who do formal meditation practice at home do so by themselves as "alone time." However, many people find it easier to practice consistently if they sit with others. Involvement of other people will help you with motivation and persistence. Try it with your spouse, a friend, in a mindfulness class, or with your ADHD support group. Have everyone share their experience—you may be surprised at the similarities as well as differences in individual reactions.

Tips on Informal Mindfulness Practice

Length: Informal mindfulness practice involves periodically remembering to bring your attention and curiosity to what is happening within you or around you. This practice can take a few seconds to several minutes and can be repeated many times throughout the day.

Posture and location: This form of mindfulness practice does not involve a special posture or location and does not feel like yet "another thing on the to-do list." Rather, it is a new way of relating to what you normally would be doing throughout the day. For example, you can bring enhanced attention to the actions of brushing your teeth, driving to work, talking to a friend, eating, or working out. In fact you can do it now: for instance, as you're reading this, become aware of your shoulders and notice any sensations present there.

Difficulties: Informal practice is easy to do but it is hard to remember to do it. Thus reminders are often helpful to beginners (for example, setting an alarm on your phone to remind you to take a deep mindful breath every two hours). With practice, tuning to the present moment becomes more automatic and spontaneous. Another difficulty that may arise is that it can be hard to be mindful in the midst of strong emotions. Step 6 discusses ways to overcome this obstacle.

Labeling Thoughts and Feelings

When we practice mindfulness, inevitably at some point our attention will wander away from the present moment. For example, we stop paying attention to our breath and instead we'll start thinking about what to make for dinner, or we'll rerun a difficult conversation we had at work that day. Labeling is a helpful tool for noting when our attention has wandered and gently bringing it back to the present.

When we label, we silently acknowledge to ourselves where our mind has gone with a word or phrase that describes our moment-by-moment experience, for example "planning," "worrying," "itching," "feeling impatient." One of the most useful labels is simply "thinking," which covers most of what pulls us away from the present moment. This can be done in the course of formal or informal practice.

Mindfulness = Perceiving or noticing

Labeling = Describing what's noticed with a word or phrase

It is important not to use labeling as a way of criticizing yourself—for example, "Gosh, I am thinking again! What's wrong with me!" Remember, *everyone's mind can wander*. The Buddhist meditation teacher Pema Chödrön instructs her students that labeling thoughts should be like touching a bubble with a feather. You gently pop the bubble and return to the breath. Use that kind of gentle touch when you notice that your mind has wandered off.

Labeling is also helpful with observing difficult thoughts or feelings. From clinical experience and brain research we know that naming emotional states can calm our nervous system and help us manage intense negative thoughts and feelings.[1] It's like the saying "If you can name it then you can tame it." When labeling difficult feelings, simply notice what's happening from a dis-identified, witnessing perspective. For example, instead of saying "I'm judgmental," you would just note "Ah, a negative judgment" or simply "judgment." Instead of saying "I'm angry," you would just use the words "oh, there is anger" or simply "anger." This helps us to step back from the thoughts or feelings we're having and just observe the mind patterns without automatically seeing them as "who we are" or "the truth" about us or the world around us.

MINDFULNESS

Again, it is a given that during mindfulness practice the mind will wander off at some point. This is true for everyone and even more common in those with ADHD. This is also an opportunity to label and get to know how your mind works. In fact, you can say that if you have ADHD, you have more opportunities to notice and label distractions. When this happens, you can simply say in your mind "wandering" or "thinking" and take a brief mental snapshot of where the mind wandered to. Then gently bring your attention back to what you intended to pay attention to.

Don't get caught up in having to label everything perfectly. Start with the obvious things like "the breath" or "thinking." As you practice, it will be easier to label more subtle levels of perception. We will also talk more about labeling difficult thoughts and emotions in steps 5 and 6 of this book.

"My ADHD": Observe Your Own Unique ADHD Patterns

I imagine some readers of this book know a lot about ADHD, and some may be just beginning to understand what ADHD means in their lives. Regardless of where you are on your ADHD journey, however, I encourage you right now to take some time to review common ADHD symptoms and ponder how ADHD is affecting your life. Such review will later help you mindfully recognize your ADHD patterns as we go through the steps.

A checklist is provided at the end of the book to aid your reflections. When reflecting on your own symptoms, strive to be nonjudgmental and compassionate. See if you can bring an investigative and nonreactive attitude. As you reflect, reframe ADHD from being a "deficit" to being a difference, an example of biological diversity. See if you can approach your own constellation of ADHD symptoms with newfound curiosity: you want to understand what is involved and you want to learn, which requires an open mind. It often helps to do such reflection with someone who knows you well, such as your spouse or a friend. Their input can point out difficulties you may not be aware of. Again, it's important that you and others reflect on your symptoms with an open mind and with compassion for each other's point of view. And if you can bring some humor to this exercise, even better!

A Mindful Review of Your ADHD Symptoms

Find the ADHD checklist on pages 206–8 and review it. As you do, ask yourself:

What is my ADHD like?

How does it manifest in my life?

Think of specific situations (such as with work or in relationships) as you answer these questions, and ask others for examples as well.

THINGS FOR YOU TO KNOW

1. Current clinical guidelines require you to have at least six out of nine symptoms in either the inattentive or impulsive/hyperactive group to meet the threshold for an ADHD diagnosis. You also have to have a history of some symptoms in childhood and experience significant difficulties in at least two important areas of your life.
2. Our thinking about adult ADHD is evolving, and new checklists that include executive function and emotional regulation symptoms are being developed. For an expanded checklist of common adult ADHD patterns, see *Taking Charge of Adult ADHD* (2010) by Dr. Russell Barkley.
3. While a checklist can help you identify some symptoms, it can't substitute for a formal assessment with a clinician. The clinician can help you make sense of your experiences and assess if other conditions or circumstances are contributing to your ADHD complaints.

Part Two

MINDFULNESS FOR ADHD

The Eight-Step Program

Introduction

This part of the book presents the eight-step program in mindfulness for ADHD. Steps 1–3 focus on strengthening your ability to move out of automatic pilot, train attention control, and focus on the present moment. Steps 4–8 show you how you can use these core mindfulness skills to observe and manage your thoughts, feelings, and actions. The steps build on each other, so it's best to do them in the order presented. I recommend spending one to two weeks exploring the specific mindfulness exercises described in each step before moving on to the next one. However, feel free to move through the steps at your own pace.

Included with this book is an audio CD that provides guided meditation instruction for selected exercises in the eight-step program. You can also download this audio program by visiting www.shambhala.com/MindfulnessPrescription.

Overview of the Steps

Step 1. Become More Present: *Attention and the Five Senses*

Step 2. Focus the Wandering Mind: *Mindful Breathing*

Step 3. Direct and Anchor Your Awareness: *Mindfulness of Sound, Breath, and Body*

Step 4. Listen to Your Body: *Mindfulness of Body Sensations and Movement*

Step 5. Observe Your Mind: *Mindfulness of Thoughts*

Step 6. Manage Your Emotions: *Mindfulness of Feelings*

Step 7. Communicate Skillfully: *Mindful Listening and Speaking*

Step 8. Slow Down to Be More Effective: *Mindful Decisions and Actions*

Become More Present

Attention and the Five Senses

Rick is always on the go and keeps shifting his attention from one thing to another. He constantly checks his BlackBerry and multitasks throughout the day. During meals he often reads the newspaper, watches TV, or both. His work computer tends to have multiple screens open as he juggles e-mail, Facebook, Twitter, and work files. When driving, he often makes business phone calls. Lately he has been feeling more scattered, stressed, and exhausted—yet he still finds it hard to unwind.

M any of us have fast-paced lives and our attention is constantly pulled in different directions. In many ways this is a sign of our times—the electronic age is upon us, offering endless information and entertainment. However, this on-the-go, distracted life is, and has always been, very common in adults with ADHD. Those like Rick, who have ADHD with hyperactivity, are driven from one task to another impulsively, often ending up with several simultaneous projects. Others, like a patient of mine named Leanne who has inattentive ADHD, are easily distracted and in this way end up doing several things at once. In the end, both Rick and Leanne often end up feeling scattered and stressed.

While reasons for being scattered may be different, the antidote is learning to *pause and shift your attention—this time in a purposeful way—to the present moment.* This shift helps us step back from being driven, distracted, or absentminded and creates a new opportunity for choice in our actions. The shift—an essential pause—ultimately becomes the braking mechanism that allows us to move out of automatic-pilot mode. As we learn to pause, we can more easily tell ourselves: "Maybe I don't have to do this in this way."

The Science of Attention

If you have ADHD, you probably tend to think about your lack of focus with frustration and discouragement: "Why can't I pay attention?!" But as we begin this first step of the eight-step program, which focuses on the fundamental pausing and shifting of attention to the present moment, I invite you to ponder attention in the way a scientist might: studying what attention is and how it is in different situations.

Scientific study of attention shows us that it is not a single mental function but a complex system with several distinct branches or networks. A prominent researcher of attention, Dr. Michael Posner at the University of Oregon, describes three attention networks: *alerting, orienting,* and *conflict* attention (also called executive attention).[1]

Alerting has to do with *readying or gearing up attention* to respond to experiences, and it also involves maintaining good alertness over time. *Vigilance* and *alert arousal* are related to this network. Think of the quality of your attention when you are interested in something, and compare that to your diminished attention when you experience something as boring or repetitive. Think about your ability to pay attention when you are rested versus when you are tired. The difference in the brightness and readiness of your attention is a difference in alerting.

Orienting has to do with *movement of attention* toward a sensory stimulus or shifting attention from one thing to another. For example, if you move your attention from one side of this page to another, you engage your orienting network. While orienting is often related to moving visual attention from one spot to another, it also includes internal shifts of attention.

Conflict attention has to do with choosing and controlling responses, and it is involved in *paying attention despite distractions*. For instance, if you choose to ignore an itching sensation and keep reading, or if you keep your focus on paying your bills despite an urge to check your e-mail, you are using your conflict-attention network.

Attention Is Like a Flashlight

A flashlight analogy is handy to get a feel for the three branches of attention: alerting is like turning the flashlight on; orienting is like pointing it toward what you want to see; and conflict attention is keeping the light in one place even if something else is distracting. Also like a flashlight, wherever you place your attention, the spot becomes illuminated and more clearly perceived.

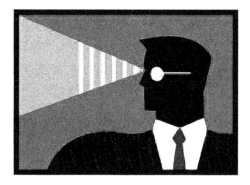

Research shows that not all attention networks are equally impaired in ADHD: the alerting and conflict attention networks are less efficient, while the orienting network is usually intact.[2]

There are other ways to describe the different aspects of

attention: *selective attention* refers to focusing on one activity or object while "tuning out" other stimuli; *divided attention* means paying attention to more than one thing; and *sustained attention* involves maintaining alert and focused attention even when it is hard to do. Some people in the field also refer to *voluntary attention* (attention that is self-directed) as being "top-down," meaning that the individual is actively directing where his or her attention is going. By contrast, *involuntary attention* (when our attention is pulled away by something) is called "bottom-up."

Attention in ADHD Life

ADHD adults often experience a whole spectrum of attention-regulation difficulties ranging from a lack of focus to trouble with shifting attention, or hyperfocus. They typically report that if something is routine or boring, paying attention comes at great effort. Complaints of having scattered attention, feeling distracted, overlooking details, and making careless mistakes are common. At the same time, novel, interesting, or exciting tasks can be very absorbing to adults with ADHD. These tasks can hold their attention, or keep them hyperfocused, for long stretches of time. Such intense focus may be an asset when working on a project, but it can also create problems in daily life. When hyperfocused, we can lose track of time, be oblivious to what's happening around us, and get stuck in the details of a project. A hyperfocused person may end up neglecting basic self-care (for example, sitting at the computer for hours despite being hungry or needing to get some rest), have trouble transitioning to another task, or ignore requests from others.

It's often said that in ADHD the problem isn't that a person isn't able to pay attention, but that he or she isn't able to pay attention *to the right thing at the right time*. Accordingly, strategies that strengthen regulation of attention and executive function—knowing how and when to sustain focus on something and how and when to shift focus to something else—are much needed in order to cope with ADHD.

Attention and Mindfulness

Mindfulness is a practice of being alert and attentive yet relaxed. This is in contrast to how we tend to pay attention in daily life: with effort, tension, and stress. Mindfulness is less about doing something with effort and more about allowing the experience to reveal itself to you. For that reason we often say mindfulness is "dropping into" awareness. Mindfulness involves both focusing on the present moment and monitoring our attention. Keep that in mind as we go through the exercises below and the rest of the eight-step program.

Mindfulness involves both focusing and monitoring our attention.

Now let's investigate different aspects of attention through several short mindful explorations.

EXPLORATION 1.1
Playing with Visual Attention and Awareness

While attention and awareness often go together, there are also times when they can exist independent of one another. For instance, when "going through the motions," we may pay attention but lack full awareness. Driving a car along a familiar route is a good example of this state of mind. By contrast, in the case of peripheral vision, we may have awareness even though there is no direct attention. With the practice of mindfulness we can start observing how attention and awareness function in our lives. We can pay attention to our awareness and be aware of our attention.

Below is a famous visual illusion called Rubin's vase[3] that demonstrates the interplay between attention and awareness.

1. What do you see when you look at this picture?

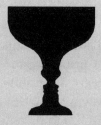

A vase?
How about two faces?
How about both the vase and the faces simultaneously?

The key here is that your awareness changes depending on where you place your attention. You can focus your attention on either the vase or the pair of faces, or you can try to see the vase and the faces at the same time. If you get fixed on one of the images, however, you can become unaware of the other one. When you fix your attention on the vase, the more prominent or attention-grabbing image, it's almost as if the faces do not exist. In our lives, we can also get "fixed" on one way of seeing things, even though multiple possibilities might exist.

2. Can you further expand your awareness by noticing the physical space between you and what you're observing? Notice how you feel when you do that.[4]

EXPLORATION 1.2
Playing with Non-Visual Attention

1. Close your eyes, or, if you prefer, keep them open with a gaze resting in one spot.
2. Notice what is coming to your awareness from the *outside*

world. You may be noticing sounds or sensing the temperature of the room.

3. Now, shift your attention to the *inside* of yourself. See what grabs your attention. For example, you can notice the contact between your body and your seat, the sensations on your face, or your breath. You may also notice a feeling or a thought.

4. Move your attention from the top of your head toward your jaw and check if you are clenching your teeth. If you notice tension in your jaw, relax the area, and notice the change in sensation. Notice how easy or difficult it is for you to focus on the outside or the inside worlds.

Rediscovering Five Senses

We now continue to practice the mindful shift from automatic pilot to the present moment by tuning our attention to our five basic senses.

1. Seeing
2. Hearing
3. Smelling
4. Tasting
5. Touching

Typically, in response to the inputs from our senses, we often automatically begin to think, compare, react, or remember. For example, if we see or hear a siren, we may start thinking of an ambulance or maybe react with some annoyance at its loudness.

The following exercise instead invites us to stay with the *direct experience of the senses*, such as noticing the sound without opinions or evaluations or comparisons. This exercise is a practice in becoming more fully present, rather than just falling into habitual reactions. In addition, focusing on the five senses can help us feel more relaxed, less driven, and more alive. It is a way of giving our mind a break.

EXPLORATION 1.3
Tuning In to the Five Senses

Imagine that you are tuning to different stations on the radio. The first station picks up a visual signal, the second one tunes to sounds, the third one to scents, the fourth one transmits taste, the fifth one touch. Let's go through the stations in sequence. Practice "just experiencing" each and keep an open attitude.

Seeing Explore your surroundings with your eyes. Notice what's around you as if you were a photographer interested in capturing interesting lines, colors, textures, and angles in your view. You may notice different judgments or thoughts about what you see, but don't get caught up in them. Simply practice "just seeing."

Hearing Tune in to the sounds around you. Bring attention to the sounds as they come and go, and note any moments of silence in between. Practice awareness of sounds without getting caught up in mental associations with each sound. If you start to analyze the sound, gently return your attention to "just hearing."

Be open even to unpleasant noises. Practice receiving familiar sounds, like a lawnmower, simply as sounds with a certain intensity or quality. If you happen to read this in a quiet space (though few are totally silent when you open your awareness to sound), you can scratch your head and notice the sound.

Smelling Notice the smells around you, paying attention to any scent or odor present. If there is no perceptible smell, note the absence of smell.

Look for opportunities in your environment to open your awareness to scents. For example, you can also bring your hand to your nose and notice if you smell anything on the back of your hand, your palm, or your fingertips; perhaps a trace of soap, or a scent of food you handled, or simply sweat. As before, refrain from thinking about the smell. Instead, practice "just smelling." You can also pick up some fruit, open a marker, or smell a flower or a plant. What the heck, pick up your shoe and smell it, too. Be creative!

Tasting Next, tune in to the sense of taste. Pick a small morsel of food, like a raisin, a grape, some chocolate, or a beverage. As you bite into the food or take a sip, note the basic quality of the taste (salty, sour, sweet, bitter, and so forth). Practice "just tasting" as if you were eating this type of food for the first time. To enhance this experience, try a food that you haven't had before.

Touching Finally, notice your sense of touch. As babies we used our hands and whole bodies to learn about the world (often together with mouthing everything we could get our hands on). See if you can explore this sense by finding different things and surfaces to touch and feel.

For example, you can bring the back of your hand to your lips and gently touch it, noticing any sensations this creates. How about touching the cover of this book and noticing its texture? Maybe you notice a feeling of smoothness or roughness, of coolness or warmth. Try pressing your finger on your thigh and exploring the sensation of pressure. Or rub your hands together and see how your palms feel afterward. For a stronger sensation, try holding an ice cube.

Sensory Input and ADHD

SENSORY OVERLOAD

On a daily basis our senses get bombarded by an array of stimulation. But if you have ADHD, even an ordinary experience like going to a busy grocery store or a neighborhood carnival can be a mind zap or an energy drain. Due to difficulties focusing and prioritizing "too much information," the experience of sensory overload can happen in ADHD.

SENSORY PROCESSING DIFFICULTIES

Some with ADHD may experience sensory overload more than just occasionally—they may have increased sensory processing difficulties. The information coming through any of the senses can feel overwhelming and provoke an unusual response. Think of the person who wears a T-shirt and can't stand the feel of a tag on their neck or someone who is intensely bothered by the slightest smells. We all have our sensory preferences and dislikes, but for some children and adults with ADHD, their sensory difficulties can interfere with daily functioning. They may experience more irritability or more fatigue. For example, it is one thing to dislike loud noise; it is another to have your hair stand on end every time the phone rings.

If you are a person with sensory processing difficulty, tuning in to the five senses is an opportunity to understand your own sensory reactivity. For example, if you are sensitive to smell, you may experience quick irritability or even anger and an urge to pull away from a scent or an odor. More smells will seem unpleasant to you, if you are a person who experiences them with extra intensity. If, however, it is hard for you to detect smells, you may find that you have to be more creative in finding different scents to observe and that more things seem neutral in their scent.

Mindfulness in Daily Life

With ADHD, the feeling of boredom and craving for novelty can come up often and easily. Tuning in to your five senses is one way to bring interest and novelty to every moment of your life—even mundane activities can feel new and interesting. With mindfulness, even eating—something we all do every day—can feel like something you've never done before.

EXPLORATION 1.4
Mindful Eating

Here we practice awareness of all five senses using food. This practice can be incorporated into one of your meals as a regular daily or weekly practice. Mindful eating can also help curb impulsive or absentminded eating, which happens all too often with ADHD.

- Find a raisin[5] (or a berry, or another small morsel of food). Pick it up and imagine you just arrived on Earth from another planet. This is the first time you are experiencing an object like this, and you're curious about it. Take some time to inspect the food. You may notice feelings of impatience or an urge to eat quickly. If so, see if you can label the feeling without acting on it.
- Put the raisin in the palm of your hand and inspect it for visual texture, color, and shape. Smell it. Touch it with your finger and feel any texture or sensation (for example, stickiness or dryness).
- Bring the raisin to your mouth and gently touch your lips with it, noticing the sensations (such as coolness or smoothness).
- Bring the raisin to your ear and notice if you hear anything. Or notice the absence of sound.
- Now put the raisin inside your mouth, slowly chew, and taste it. Notice the movement of your jaw and tongue. Notice the sounds of eating. Notice the act of swallowing.
- Bring awareness to the fact that your body is now one raisin heavier.

Noticing Your Reactions Nonjudgmentally

During a presentation for a local ADHD support group, I led a mindful eating exercise like the one described here. After the exercise, several people, none with prior mindfulness exposure, shared their experience. One woman, Linda, commented how interesting and flavorful the raisin was compared to raisins she had eaten in the past: "I did not know that raisins have so many different grooves and colors!" she said. "And the taste of this one raisin seemed more intense than what I normally notice." She also reported becoming more relaxed just by slowing down to do the exercise.

Matt, a businessman in his mid-forties, said he hated the exercise. "My mind kept going away from the raisin to my work," he said. "I felt restless. I tried to go back to the raisin, but after a while I just wanted to quit." I told him that even though the exercise had a different effect on him than it had on Linda, it was great that he was able to notice what was happening. I asked him if he could be curious about these reactions and not judge them as good or bad. Could he explore the feelings of impatience, frustration, and restlessness a little more? Could he notice how these feelings manifest in his body? Could he also notice the feelings with compassion and continue to observe them with curiosity?

Suggested Reminders for Practice

When you first learn to practice mindfulness, you quickly come to realize that focusing on the present is generally easy—anyone can do it when prompted—but *remembering* to focus on the present is not. So why not use some reminders?

Mindfulness is about focusing our attention on the present moment *and remembering to come back to the present moment* when we become distracted.

Typically, ADHD adults are no strangers to reminders. Because their executive-function difficulties make it hard for

MINDFULNESS FOR ADHD

them to remember tasks or appointments, many adults with ADHD intuitively develop some way of reminding themselves what they need to do. They keep notes on the calendar, call themselves to leave reminder messages, make voice memos, leave Post-its all around, and even resort to the good old technique of writing notes on the palm of their hands.

In general, writing things down and posting them in a place you are likely to notice them is a great help. However, leaving loose pieces of paper all around or having haphazard reminders in multiple places—which adults with ADHD tend to do—is *not* helpful.

Here are several ways to create reminders for your mindfulness practice.

- Make an appointment in your schedule book for a mindful break: for example, five minutes of silent breath-awareness practice or mindful eating.
- Set pop-up reminders on your phone or computer that prompt you to stop and do a short mindfulness practice such as noticing your present-moment experience with your five senses.
- Use a smartphone application to help you pause and practice mindful awareness throughout the day. There are several available that are designed for mindfulness practice. Just search for "mindfulness" in your phone's app store.
- Get a mindfulness buddy (just like an exercise buddy) and text each other reminders from time to time to tune in to the present moment.
- Use a visual reminder such as a small image or sign. Post this in a place you're likely to notice it, such as on your bathroom mirror, above your desk, or on your refrigerator. The sign could say:

    ○ Where is my attention right now?
    ○ Tune into five senses
    ○ See, hear, smell, taste, touch

Step 1 at a Glance

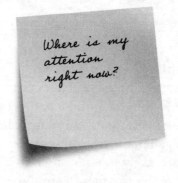

Formal Practices

- Mindful eating can be done as a formal practice. For this week, every day (or as many days as you can) eat an entire meal mindfully. Eat in silence, more slowly than usual, and notice all the sounds, tastes, smells, thoughts, and feelings that are present.
- If you eat most meals with your family, trying eating in silence for the first three to five minutes of the meal. With children, feel free to make it fun and playful.

Mindful Awareness in Daily Life

- Do an "attention check-in," setting an alarm or using a posted reminder sign. Notice what you're attending to at that moment.
- Practice shifting your attention to your senses and the present moment. For example:
    - See and touch your pet with a full awareness.
    - Smell the soap and feel the water when taking a shower.
    - Hear the sounds of traffic outside your window.
    - Cook new foods.
    - Do some gardening paying special attention to the sensations of touch and smell.
    - Experience your partner through your senses.

STEP 2 Focus the Wandering Mind

Mindful Breathing

Peter settled into his airplane seat and pulled out his book. He'd been interested in martial arts for a while and was eager to read about the history of karate. He started reading, but at some point he realized that his mind had been wandering off while his eyes kept moving over the words on the page. He didn't remember a thing about what he'd just read. He noticed he'd been thinking about his motorcycle that needed repairs, instead of the book's topic. "C'mon, focus, focus!" Peter said to himself. He backtracked to the beginning of the second chapter, and began reading again.

We've all had the experience of reading a book or a magazine story and having our mind wander somewhere else as we do so. It's as if our mind has a mind of its own! Our eyes follow and process the words on some level, but most of our attention and awareness is wrapped up in pondering something else. We end up missing pages of important information and feeling unfocused and ineffective.

The experience of a wandering mind followed by frustration is universal, but it's more frequent with ADHD. In this step of the program we focus on the breath as a way to curb a wandering mind and train our attention.

The Importance of the Breath

Let's ponder the breath for a bit. Breathing is something we do every day, but we may not realize its power as a tool for developing focus and self-regulation. Here are two key points about breath awareness.

Our Breath Is Always in the Present

The mind can go to the past, present, or future—but our breathing is always happening in the present. Focusing on the breath can therefore keep us alert and anchored to "the now." Over time, the practice of focusing (and refocusing) on the breath strengthens our ability to resist the pull of a wandering mind.

Our Breath Is the Door to Changing Our Mind-Body State

Our breathing happens automatically throughout the day. Luckily for us—imagine having to consciously direct each breath. We could scarcely do anything else. And what if you got distracted? Having ADHD would mean constantly having to catch your breath.

At the same time, breathing (like attention) is one of those things where in addition to automatic regulation, we also have the ability to consciously intervene. We can change the rate and depth of our breathing at will, by taking a deeper breath whenever we want to.

This provides a great opportunity for us to consciously shift our body physiology from "stressed" and "reactive" to "relaxed" and "stable." For example, anxiety and stress make us breathe shallowly and more through the chest. But a relaxed state often leads to deeper, belly breathing. This also works in the reverse: if we practice belly breathing, we can *induce* the relaxation response.

EXPLORATION 2.1
Noting the Breath in Three Places

You can be aware of your breathing in three basic spots:

- Nostrils
- Chest
- Belly

Explore each of these spots and see how easy or difficult it is for you to notice the breath there. You can do this with your eyes open or closed, but closing your eyes tends to help focus on the inner sensations.

Nostrils

Focus on the area around and just below your nostrils. You may notice a sensation of subtle movement, tickling, or coolness. If you find it hard to feel the breath here, put an index finger under your nose and feel the air on your finger.

Chest

Focus on the rising and falling of the rib cage for several breaths. You can also put one of your hands on your chest and sense the movement through your hand. Explore breathing through your chest by exaggerating the movement of your upper chest and shoulders. Notice how you feel.

Belly

Focus on the rising and falling of your lower abdomen. Place your hand on your belly to help you feel the movement. Imagine that you are inflating a balloon below your belly button. Notice how you feel. Finally, put one hand on your chest and one on your lower abdomen. Breathe naturally, and notice if you tend to breathe more through your chest or your belly.

Note: If you tend to be a habitual "chest breather"—a trait linked to anxiety and stress—breathing through your belly may feel unnatural at first, so don't force it. See if you can first observe your breath as it comes out naturally, then gradually shift to belly breathing.

EXPLORATION 2.2
Mindful Breathing (CD track 2; five minutes)

In this first formal meditation practice you'll be training yourself to focus and monitor your attention toward sensations of the breath. In the process, you'll also learn to catch yourself when distracted.

The accompanying CD's track 2, titled "Mindful Breathing," guides you through this practice. Listen to it at least once, as being guided is different from doing it on your own. In my experience, some people really like using a CD, but others find it monotonous after hearing it several times. So below I also outline the practice, and you can use this page as a quick reference.

- Find a relaxed and comfortable sitting position, either on the floor using a meditation cushion (or regular pillows) or in a chair.
- Keep your back upright but relaxed, as if you're sitting in a posture of dignity. Place your hands on your lap.
- Set an intention, such as: "I'm going to practice focusing on my breath right now."
- Take a deep breath and allow yourself to simply "rest in the present moment." Let your usual preoccupations or a need to do something else fall into the background.
- Focus on your breath in one spot—at your nostrils, chest, or belly.

- Bring your full attention to your breath. Notice the natural flow of air coming in and going out.
- If you notice that your mind has wandered—such as to sounds outside or to your thoughts—that's OK. Simply gently remind yourself of your intention and return to the breath.
- If your mind wanders off one hundred times, gently bring it back one hundred times.
- Practice being kind to yourself. Don't judge your experience as good or bad; simply be curious about how your mind works.
- At the end of this meditation, offer yourself some appreciation for taking the time to pause, for training your attention and awareness, and for connecting more fully with yourself in the present moment.

Mindfulness is just as much about *returning* to the breath as *staying* with the breath. This returning, or re-shifting of attention, counteracts the mind's natural tendency to wander and trains awareness and focus.

Common Difficulties in Sitting Practice

What if my mind wanders a lot?

First of all, it's OK—just bring yourself back. This is also an opportunity to notice whether you tend to be overly judgmental or critical of yourself. For example, do you start to think, "What's wrong with me, I can't even focus for five minutes?!" Try to let go of these types of negative judgments and gently return your attention to your breath. Realizing that our attention has wandered off and returning to the breath is, in fact, one of the most valuable aspects of sitting meditation practice.

If you find that your mind wanders a lot during the five minutes of sitting, there are some remedies: namely, *giving your active mind something extra to do while you continue paying attention to the breath.*

Here some suggestions:

- In your mind, repeat the words "breathing in" and "breathing out."
- Count silently, from one to ten, while you breathe, then repeat. Below are different ways of saying the numbers as you inhale and exhale:

BREATHING IN	BREATHING OUT
One...	Twooo...
Threee...	Four...
(up to ten, then repeat)	

One, two, three, four, five	Six, seven, eight, nine, ten
(repeat, starting at one)	

- When you feel more settled, you can stop counting and just notice your breath.
- Instead of counting, repeat a word that helps you slow down, feel calmer, or become present. For example, words like "relax," "peace," "calm," "it's OK," or "present." You can also use a word or phrase that has a spiritual meaning to you.
- Use a mental picture together with (or instead of) counting or repeating a word. For example, imagine a wave of air going in and out of your body as you breathe and count.

What if I get restless or sleepy?

If you find yourself restless, take a moment to observe the sensation. How do you know you're restless? How does it feel in your body? Do you notice any particular thoughts or feelings, or an urge to shift or move?

Can you challenge yourself to stay with those sensations and thoughts a little longer (are you willing to study the discomfort a little more)? Restlessness is like a wave you can surf. See if you can watch it rise up, crest, then eventually recede. Such imagery and shifts in perspective can help you tolerate the discomfort.

You can also decide to do something subtle to release the restlessness (like taking several deep breaths or changing your position). If you make a move, you can still continue to be mindful and observe shifts in your body, thoughts, and feelings. In this way, you don't have to react out of restlessness—you can learn from it or learn to just be with it.

If you find that you're still too wound up to sit still, your body may not be ready. You may need to do some vigorous physical exercise first to expend the energy. Or you may start with brisk, mindful walking, then gradually shift to slower walking until you feel ready to try sitting practice.

If you notice some sleepiness, straighten your back or open your eyes to increase your alertness. If sitting practice just makes you too sleepy, try mindful movement instead. Or do some physical activity first to increase your energy level. The sitting meditation practice may feel similar to sitting in a lecture hall for a while: it may be hard not to nod off. If that happens, it helps to stand up and stretch to get yourself awake again.

....

A friend of mine who is a rather hyper, restless person wanted to learn to meditate to curb his high blood pressure. After several unsuccessful attempts to meditate at home, he started to meditate after a gym workout, while sitting in a steam room. The physical exertion and subsequent heat of the steam helped his body to relax, making it easier for him to rest silently and focus on his breathing for ten to fifteen minutes.

....

What if there's noise or other distractions?

As you practice, you may also notice noises and other distractions, and that may be irritating. See if for a moment you can bring your attention to them and try to notice them nonjudgmentally. For example, "noises" are simply sounds that perhaps evoke an unpleasant feeling. Once you acknowledge the distraction and the feeling it provokes, see if you can return to your practice. Initially, you can also experiment using earplugs, which can help you focus more on the sound of your breath and your body sensations.

What if my mind is preoccupied by something?

If your mind is repeatedly drawn to an idea, song, image, or feeling as you sit, just continue to label your thoughts as you notice them. Practice letting go of the distraction while you *keep most of your awareness on your breathing*. The good news is that you don't have to struggle to empty your mind to practice mindfulness: you can simply be mindfully aware of what is—even the seemingly incessant chatter of the mind.

What if an uncomfortable thought or feeling comes up?

See if you can accept and label it (for example, "anger" or "fear"). If the feeling is a significant physical or emotional pain, try opening yourself to it gently and noticing its sensations for a moment. Then shift your attention to a place that feels safe or comfortable, such as your breath, your palms, or a calming phrase or image. You can work with the painful feeling by moving your attention back and forth between the pain and a safe or comfortable place. (See steps 4 through 6 for more on working with difficult feelings.)

What if I start feeling bored or doubt I should be doing meditation?

If you notice boredom or doubting, don't judge these feelings as bad; instead, acknowledge and label them (for instance, "boredom feeling," "doubting thought"), and bring attention back to what you originally set out to do. You can also remind yourself of your motivation for what you're doing and thereby reframe it from being an unpleasant task to being a new learning experience and an act of self-care. See if you can become re-inspired to explore awareness, and notice how your mind and body states change from moment to moment. You can also explore what a feeling of boredom is really like: for example, what do you notice in your body, your energy level, or your attitude when you're bored?

Kathy's First Try

Kathy had been reading about mindfulness training and its positive effects on attention and emotions. She was very motivated to start the eight-week course. In the first class session she learned about the basic breath-awareness practice and was eager to do the five-minute exercise at home. She planned to do the practice the next morning, but found she "ran out of time" and had to leave for work.

The next day, she made a point to do it at lunch in a nearby park. As she practiced, she found that her mind wandered a lot. She tried again at home and found herself questioning if she was doing it right. At the next class, she complained, "I'm a failure at this; my mind won't stop." She was reassured that a wandering mind is a universal experience and part of mindfulness practice, and that it is also much more common with ADHD. She was encouraged to simply be curious about her experience—whatever it is—and practice "returning to the breath." That helped her relax and not criticize herself for "failing at mindfulness."

She found that as her mindfulness class progressed, she could do five or more minutes of practice on most days, and if she missed several days, she was able to return to it again. While not every practice period proved to be calming or easy, over time she felt more centered and focused during her sitting meditation periods and in daily life.

EXPLORATION 2.3
Mindful Breathing and Walking (five minutes)

If restlessness makes it difficult to sit, you can also practice awareness of the breath while walking. You can do this practice indoors or out. When doing the meditation indoors, you don't need a lot of space—you can simply find a small area and practice walking in a straight line, then turning and walking back along the same line.

- Walk slowly with your eyes open and softly focused a short distance in front of you. (Avoid looking around, as it can be distracting; however, keep yourself aware of where you're going.)
- Focus on sensations of the breath as you slowly walk. If you like, synchronize your breathing with your footsteps. For example, as you step with your right foot, you can inhale, and as you step with your left foot, you can exhale.

Mindful Breathing in Daily Life

You can incorporate mindfulness into your daily life simply by remembering to notice the breath, even for a few seconds, in the midst of your usual activities. For example:

- As you're reading this, simply notice your breath.
- Sense the rising and falling of your belly as you breathe in and out.
- Notice the pause between the in-breath and the out-breath.
- Do this for a few breaths and then decide to either return to reading or take a break from reading.

Mindful breathing is a powerful way to connect more fully with what you're doing in each moment. It also creates a conscious choice. Another good practice is taking one deep, conscious breath before starting an activity. Even one breath can make a difference in how focused and aware you feel, and can change the rest of your experience. For example, take a deep breath before reading each chapter of this book, dialing your phone, or before talking with your boss. Try it and see how it feels for you.

Suggested Reminders for Practice

- Bring attention to your breathing throughout your day. At the top of your to-do list, write "Breath" or "Breathe Before You Start." As you tackle the tasks on your list, periodically take a breath with awareness.
- Use visual reminders: place them in your work area, on the fridge, or anywhere you're likely to see them. This could be a simple sign by your workspace or telephone that says "Breathe."

....

Step 2 at a Glance

Formal Practice

Do five minutes of mindful breathing each day (CD track 2).

Mindful Awareness in Daily Life

- Use visual reminders or set an alarm on your phone to remind you to stop and take a deep mindful breath from time to time. (If you can, set your alarm to go off every one to two hours.)
- Try mindful walking and breathing on the way to or from work or when doing errands.

STEP 3 Direct and Anchor Your Awareness

Mindfulness of Sound, Breath, and Body

Lucy has often been described as "spacey." When she was younger, her mom used to call her "D.D. Girl," short for "daydreaming girl." She remembers often drifting in and out of awareness while listening to her elementary school teacher. Her mind would wander and roam until something snapped her out of it.

As an adult, Lucy continues to daydream a lot. Recently, while talking to her friends about a park in LA, Lucy started wondering about her aunt in New Jersey. Why? Because going to a park made her think of bringing her red blanket, which reminded her of going to college in New York (she used the blanket in her dorm), which in turn made her remember that she needs to call her aunt in New Jersey.

This zigzag movement of attention can happen quickly and easily for Lucy, and it can make her miss out on actual conversations taking place. On the flip side, Lucy has a great imagination and has written several short stories that were published by a local magazine. She credits her daydreaming as the best time to come up with good story ideas.

If you have inattentive ADHD, Lucy's experience will probably resonate with you. In this step, we'll use mindfulness to explore the dance—the movements and shifts—of awareness and focus to help curb excessive daydreaming. You will practice "sitting in the driver's seat" of your ADHD mind and guiding it to the present moment. Later on, in step 5, we'll look at "mindful daydreaming" as a tool for insight and creativity.

Movement of Attention and Awareness

As you've probably already noticed, attention and awareness have a natural tendency to move. This movement is particularly obvious or noticeable as we listen to music. Music is a collection of different sounds with changing tempo and intensity, and listening to it involves shifting awareness from one note, instrument, or tempo to another. Listening to music also involves anticipating certain changes and sustaining attention. Neuroimaging studies show that listening to music is a good way to activate the brain networks involved in paying attention.[1] As it turns out, our attention is especially stimulated by the short pauses between musical movements as we anticipate the next note.

So let's observe how attention and awareness move in response to musical patterns. When listening to music you have a choice in how you pay attention. You can listen intently to the changes in the sounds (focused attention) or you can allow the sounds to come and go (open attention).

EXPLORATION 3.1
Listening to Music

- Choose a piece of instrumental music such as classical, jazz, or world music. (When starting out, it helps to pick an instrumental piece—that is, with no singing—as listening for words may make it difficult to stay with the experience of sounds. Later on you can try this exercise with any music and compare your experience.)
- Sitting silently with your eyes closed or slightly open (whichever is most comfortable for you), start listening to the music.

- Notice any shifts in the music's tempo or intensity, and listen to the different sounds. As you listen, notice what happens to your attention and awareness. Also notice the following:
    - Is the music evoking certain feelings, thoughts, or imagery for you?
    - Does the music influence your body? Is there an urge to move?
- Continue listening and noticing thoughts, feelings, and body sensations until the music ends.

It's fun to do this exercise in a group and have everybody share their experience afterward. You'll find that the same music has different effects on different people. Also, experiment with music you like and don't like; for example, when you're in a car, change the channels on the radio and note your reaction to jazz, rock, classical, or country music.

Q: I often use music to relax during my meditation; it puts me in a "zone" that makes me feel calmer. Am I still practicing mindful awareness?

In typical mindfulness practice we strive to be alert and aware of what's happening in the present moment. This is different from meditations that get into a state of being absorbed by the experience or "in the zone." Getting in the zone can be more like daydreaming than being aware and alert. Our intention in practicing mindfulness is not to feel calm but to train our focus and alertness. When we listen to music, we're listening for the moment-to-moment changes and shifts in the sound rather than being "swept up by the music."

At the same time, it helps to be relaxed when we do formal mindfulness practice. If you find that music really helps you unwind, it's fine to use it in that way at the beginning of your meditation. You can also practice maintaining some awareness even as you allow yourself to be relaxed by the music. Once you feel calm, you can then decide to notice the dance of sounds, moment by moment, or focus on other aspects of your meditation, for instance, the breath.

Matching Attention with Intention

Imagine you're in a conference session. You intend to listen to the speaker, but your mind takes you elsewhere. That's not a bad thing if the talk is boring and you want a mental escape, but what if you really are interested and *want* to pay attention? Then the wandering mind can be frustrating. One way to curb daydreaming is to develop *a habit of matching your attention with a previously set intention*. You can do this by asking yourself:

- Where is my attention right now?
- Is it matching my previous intention?

We explore this in the following formal meditation practice.

EXPLORATION 3.2
Mindfulness of Sound, Breath, and Body (CD track 3; ten minutes)

With this exercise, you set an intention to pay attention to a specific thing—either sounds in your environment, your breath, or your body sensations—all of which anchor you to the present moment. You practice staying with (or returning to) the anchor until you consciously decide to pick another one. This puts you in the "driver's seat of your attention" and strengthens your ability to make transitions in your focus. The CD guides and paces you through the meditation. If you choose to do it on your own, it helps to set the timer for three-minute intervals as described below. Choose an alarm that is gentle or quiet to avoid being startled by its ring.

- Find your meditation posture (sitting upright in a chair or on a pillow). You can also do this practice while walking slowly. Take a few deep breaths to relax before you begin.
- *Set the intention to notice sounds.* For example, silently say to yourself "I'm going to notice sounds." Set your timer for three minutes.
    - Bring awareness to sounds around you. If you're indoors, notice sounds inside the room as well as outside of it.
    - Allow each sound to come to you without "reaching" for it; simply note its coming and going without getting caught up in a story about what each sound is or why it's there.
    - Whenever you notice that your attention has wandered off, briefly label it as "wandering" or "daydreaming," then gently return your attention to sound.
    - Continue this for three minutes in silence until your timer goes off.
- Now, *set the intention to notice your breath* and start your timer for another three minutes.
    - Gently rest your attention on the sensations of your breathing (at your nostrils, your chest, or your abdomen).
    - Observe the breath in its natural flow.
    - Again, whenever you notice that your attention has wandered, briefly label it as "wandering" or "daydreaming," then gently return to your breath.
    - Continue this for three minutes or so in silence.
- Now, *set the intention to notice all body sensations.* Start your timer for the next three minutes.
    - Bring attention to your body and sense it sitting. Notice the points of contact with your seat and the sense of weight resting there.
    - Explore the body from the inside. There might be a

feeling of pressure or tightness somewhere, itching or tingling, discomfort or pain. You may also notice the urge to move, or general restlessness. Notice whatever is present with curiosity.

- ○ You may notice your attention jumping from sensation to sensation, or being grabbed by a particularly strong sensation.
- ○ Again, whenever you notice that your attention has wandered away from body sensations, briefly label it as "wandering" or "daydreaming," then gently return your attention to your body.
- ○ Continue this for three minutes or so in silence.
- End your meditation by offering yourself some appreciation for sitting through this practice and directing your attention with enhanced awareness.

Q: I find it hard to focus on only one thing. It seems like I can hear the hum of the fan, notice my breath, and feel my foot itching all at the same time. It's as if my attention has different channels all at once.

If that's your experience, I recommend thinking of *foreground* and *background* awareness. If you've chosen to focus on sound, practice keeping sounds in the foreground of your awareness and allow other things to fall into the background. When it's time to focus on other things, like breath, then let the sounds fall into the background.

Step 3 in Daily Life: The Three Anchors of Mindfulness

Think of sounds, breath, and body sensations as your three main mindfulness anchors. No matter where you are and what you're doing, you can easily tune in to one or all of these anchors with mindfulness, even for few seconds. There are often some sounds in the environment (or you can notice silence)—and your breath and body are always available.

THREE ANCHORS TO THE PRESENT: SOUND, BREATH, BODY

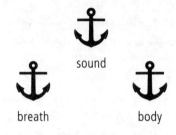

sound

breath   body

EXPLORATION 3.3
The STOP Practice

The following STOP exercise is another way to help you practice mindfulness in daily life. No matter where you are in your day, you can use STOP to become more aware of the present moment.

S = Stop (or pause)
T = Take a breath and relax
O = Observe in the present moment
- What sounds do I notice?
- What is my breath like right now?
- How does my body feel right now?
P = Proceed
- Where was my attention before STOP, and did it match my intention?
- Do I continue what I'm doing, or do something else?

Let's try it:

- Stop, take a deep breath, and relax. For a few seconds, notice the sounds around you.
- Next, notice your breathing with curiosity. If it feels shallow, breathe more deeply and through your belly.

- Move your attention to your body and notice how it feels right now. Do you notice a general sense of energy or tiredness? Are there any other sensations present? If you notice areas of tension, practice relaxing your body.
- Now remember what you were doing just before STOP-ing. Was your mind wandering or were you distracted? If so, try renewing your focus on your intention.

STOP is an all-purpose practice that we can use as a way of turning on a mindful perspective. Here we use this practice to connect with and observe the three anchors. In later steps, we will expand this practice to gradually include observation of thoughts, feelings, and actions.

STOP as a Visual Reminder

Lucy wanted to curb her spaceyness and decided to use the STOP practice to notice sounds, her breath, or her body sensations throughout her day. Sometimes she focused on one of these anchors at a time, and sometimes she decided to have her attention dance between them. She posted signs saying STOP in her bedroom, bathroom, and living room. Each night before going to bed, Lucy would make it a point to notice her breath, putting her hand on her stomach for a while. The practice also became a reminder for her to start the transition to go to sleep.

In the bathroom, the STOP sign was a cue for Lucy to pay attention to the sensations and sounds of brushing her teeth, washing her face, and taking a shower—instead of doing these activities on autopilot.

In the living room, Lucy made a point to tune in to sounds from time to time. Noises from outside gave her plenty of opportunity for a mini STOP practice. She found that doing this short exercise made her feel more connected with herself and everything she was doing.

Once, when she was engrossed in reading a magazine, a sound grabbed her attention and reminded her of mindfulness practice. She noticed a feeling of reluctance to stop reading, but decided to pause for the STOP practice. For a few seconds she tuned in to hearing sounds with full awareness. Doing this lessened the grip of her hyperfocus on reading and also made her more aware that she had intended to pay a bill and then go out. She put down the magazine and moved on to those tasks.

Suggested Reminders for Practice

Post signs in your home or workplace, such as:

- Attention and intention check-in
- Three Anchors: Sounds, Breath, Body
- STOP (Stop, Take a breath, Observe, Proceed)

Step 3 at a Glance

Formal Practice

- Do ten minutes of sound-breath-body meditation each day (as a sitting or a walking meditation).

Mindful Awareness in Daily Life

- Listen to music with mindfulness.
- Practice STOPing.
- Seek out opportunities for an enhanced sense of sound, breath, or body. For example:
  - Notice your breath and body after exercise.
  - Take a walk in nature and notice sounds around you; be aware of your breath and body during your walk. (The website www.peacefulwalks.com simulates the sounds of being in nature; try it when you're stuck at home or work.)

STEP 4   Listen to Your Body

Mindfulness of Body Sensations and Movement

Jack is frequently restless. In grade school, he'd get up out of his seat more than the other kids, he'd run around, and consequently he'd get reprimanded by his teacher. As an adult, he feels a lot of twitchy, nervous energy that drives him to constantly be in motion. He says that sitting in a work meeting feels like "endless torture," and he takes a lot of work breaks to ease his restlessness.

Adults with ADHD often have a complicated relationship to their bodies. Frequently it is a relationship of frustration or neglect. Those with hyperactivity can feel aggravated at their restlessness and look for ways to diffuse it. Those with inattention can be frustrated at their lack of energy and sluggishness. Some struggle with clumsiness. Many adults with ADHD are also impulsive, distracted, or overly committed and end up neglecting basic self-care like eating, sleeping, or having doctor's checkups. Finally, some abuse their bodies through reckless physical activity or addictions.

In this step we'll focus on developing a curious and kind relationship with the body by exploring mindfulness of physical sensations and of movement. You will learn to listen to your body and to work with difficult sensations like restlessness, low energy, muscle tension, or pain. Mindfulness of the body will also pave the way for steps 5 and 6, working with difficult emotions and thoughts.

Learning to Listen to the Body

Mary always seems to be rushing. Her days are often spent doing a thousand little things and running out of time. Even though she's already overwhelmed, she keeps taking on new commitments. When she arrives at my office for a therapy session, I first ask her to just sit quietly and notice her breathing. After few minutes, she lets out a sigh, saying, "I am so tired." By slowing down even for this brief respite, she notices how exhausted she is. "What is your body telling you?" I ask. "I really need to rest—I'm doing too much," she says with sadness. Her body had a message for her, but in the midst of her busyness the message was lost. Mary needed to start paying fuller attention to her body and taking better care of herself. Otherwise, she risked developing chronic stress problems.

Driven by life's demands and a multitude of distractions—new projects, appointments, the Internet, or other people—adults with ADHD like Mary often ignore what is happening inside of them. Signals from the body such as fatigue, pain, or tension are pushed aside. Yet the body has important messages for us, if we'd only learn to pay full attention to them.

The body is the source of deep self-knowledge. Sometimes before we fully realize something consciously, our bodies are already registering or expressing it in some way. Messages from our body may take the form of an inner restlessness felt days before a sad anniversary or stomach knots when going to work. It may also be a tingling energy before going on a date or a sense of ease when doing something we are good at.

By using mindfulness to focus on body sensations, we can access a valuable or healing message. Thus mindfulness leads to a fully embodied life—one in which our mind and body are aligned and communicating with each other.

....

The body often has important messages for us if we'd only pay full attention to it.

....

EXPLORATION 4.1
Body Scan (CD track 4; twelve minutes)

The body scan is a powerful tool for aligning mind, body, and heart. This mindfulness practice involves listening to the body by sequentially focusing on different regions of the body and noting whatever sensations are present there.[1]

In a typical body scan, a person moves her attention slowly from head to toe until the whole body is "scanned." If it helps, you can imagine your body with a grid pattern dividing it into specific sections: front versus back, right versus left, top versus bottom. You can scan these sections in any order that's comfortable for you.

BODY PLANES

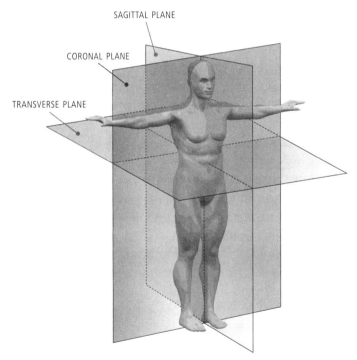

SAGITTAL PLANE

CORONAL PLANE

TRANSVERSE PLANE

ILLUSTRATION BY YASSINE MRABET

While you can do a body scan either lying down (on your back) or sitting down, the pull of gravity you experience when lying down can help you relax the body and notice sensations more easily. However you may find that it is harder for you to stay awake or that your mind wanders a lot in this position. (In fact, some people with sleep problems find that doing a body scan lying in bed helps them to fall asleep.) But if your intention is to train yourself in body awareness and relaxation in the midst of your daily life, then either sitting up or performing the practice lying down when fully awake is best. Track 4 on the CD guides you through the body scan, and here is the sequence:

- Find your position, either sitting upright or lying down on your back. Use pillows and blankets to make yourself feel comfortable and supported (for example, using pillows under your head, neck, and knees).
- Take a few deep breaths and let your body relax. Close your eyes, or keep them half-closed and resting in one spot.
- Imagine that your attention is like a flashlight, and you are pointing your attention at each section of the body to illuminate it.

TOP AND FRONT OF HEAD
- Start by focusing on the top of your head. Can you feel any sensations there: maybe an itching, vibration, or tightness? Or maybe there's no sensation at all. Whatever you notice, label it in your mind: for example, "tingling."
- Move your attention to your forehead. Pause to see if there's any sensation, and relax any areas of tension.
- Move your attention to your eyes and relax them.
- Moving down your face, notice your cheeks and your nose. There may be a slight sensation of air moving in and out of your nostrils.

- Direct your attention to your mouth and jaw, and soften the muscles around them.
- Notice your chin and the front of your throat, and if needed, relax them.

BACK OF YOUR HEAD
- Move your attention around to the back of your head and neck and notice any sensations there.
- If there is any sense of holding or tension, relax your neck.

RIGHT SHOULDER AND ARM
- Bring your attention to your right shoulder. Is there anything to feel there? Scan the front and back of it. If there's any tension, relax your shoulders.
- Move your attention down to your upper right arm. Investigate for a moment.
- Notice any sensations around your elbow.
- Move your attention to the lower arm, then your wrist and hand.
- Feel all five fingers. Slightly stretch or move your fingers and notice the sensations.

....

As you scan, notice any feelings of impatience, wanting to rush, or any other thoughts that arise. Label them—for example, "impatience"—then return to the scanning process. In this way you are also practicing patience.

....

LEFT SHOULDER AND ARM
- Slowly repeat the previous sequence but now for the left shoulder and arm, working your way down from your upper arm to your elbow, then your wrist and your left hand.

BACK

- Move your attention to your upper back and scan for any sensations there. If you're lying down you may notice points of contact with whatever you're lying on (floor or bed) and a sense of pressure.
- Scan your attention across your upper back and then down your spine to your lower back. Notice what is there, and relax any areas of tension.

CHEST

- Move your attention to the chest and feel the sensations there. There may be a slight movement up and down with each breath cycle.
- Relax your chest.

BELLY AND BETWEEN HIPS

- Notice your belly and any movement there as you breathe.
- Sense your hips on each side of the belly and notice any sensations in the pelvic area.
- Relax your hips and buttocks.

RIGHT LEG

- Now move your attention to your right leg and notice the front and the back of your thigh.
- Move to the knee. Notice any sensations in or around it.
- Next, move your attention to your calf and then your ankle.
- Notice your foot and all five toes. If you don't sense your toes, acknowledge the lack of sensations. You can also wiggle your toes and notice that.

LEFT LEG

- Repeat the previous sequence, starting with the left thigh, down toward the knee, then the calf and the foot.

WHOLE BODY

- When you're done with your left leg, open your awareness so that it includes your whole body. Are there any parts of the body or sensations that stand out for you? Notice how you feel in this moment.

Pointers on the Body Scan

1. You can start with your head and work your way toward your toes, or vice versa. In fact you can start anywhere and keep the sequence the same every time, or vary it from time to time to make it novel.

2. A variation is an "active body scan" — a practice in which you move most body parts slightly as you scan. These movement help you notice the body sensations (we did this above when feeling the fingers). For example, you can pucker your lips or smile to feel your lips. Or you can gently rotate the shoulder, arm, and wrist while you observe the sensations there.

3. If you're having trouble relaxing each body part as you scan, a similar technique called "progressive muscle relaxation" can help. In this technique you first tense the observed areas on both sides (for instance, you tighten your fists or tense your calves) and then release them for a pronounced sensation of relaxation.

4. You can also imagine that your attention is like a caring touch, a loving attention. So wherever you place your attention during the scan, in addition to noticing sensations, let an intention of caring about yourself and your body also infuse the area.

5. As you note each body area, you also can imagine that you are "breathing into it," as if you're providing fresh air to each corner of your body. Imagine that the breath helps each area relax, open up, and release any stress.

The Body Scan in Daily Life

Kelly, a graduate student, has her dissertation due in two weeks. She mapped out a schedule to work on it uninterrupted for three hours every morning. However, one morning her aunt called with news that Kelly's uncle was sick. She also wanted Kelly to look up some medical information for her. Kelly was eager to help out, but she also felt an inner tension at being pulled away from her planned schedule.

When Kelly finally returned to her dissertation a couple of hours later, she was unable to concentrate. She felt stressed by her deadline and the morning's unexpected delay. She felt a knot in her stomach, a buzzing in her body, and she was unfocused. She decided to take few minutes to sit quietly and do a body scan. As she did, she labeled what she was noticing, like "neck tension," "buzzing feeling," "restlessness," and "fast breathing." Whenever she noticed tension she took a deep breath and imagined "breathing into the area and relaxing it." After a few moments she noticed a softening in her body—a kind of tiredness but also relaxation. She sat and focused on her body until she felt more settled and ready to start writing.

ADHD and Clumsiness

As a child, Lily had been "a klutz." She remembers spilling her drink so many times as a youngster that once, highly embarrassed about knocking down her juice at breakfast, she hid in the garden for hours. As an adult, she continues to be clumsy and often bumps into others. Her husband has noticed that her sense of space and coordination skills are off. When walking together, she tends to lean toward him. When they are working together in the kitchen, he worries that she is going to back into something hot or bump her head on an open cabinet door.

At first Lily was defensive when her husband made remarks about her coordination problem—she didn't like feeling like a klutz. But with time she developed some distance from the feeling of embarrassment and her self-judgmental attitude, and she started to observe her movements with curiosity and a non-judgmental attitude. She became more aware of her body and thus more able to correct her clumsiness—for example, catching herself before she spilled a drink on her friend. Importantly, she was also more compassionate toward herself and able to respond with humor when clumsiness still led her to trip or knock something over.

In ADHD coordination and clumsiness can be a problem. Indeed, slow reaction times and difficulties with appropriate timing of movements appear more common in ADHD children and adolescents than in their non-ADHD peers.[2] Neuroimaging studies of people with ADHD show abnormalities in parts of the brain involved in movement and timing.[3]

With this knowledge and the following exercises, you can start bringing a nonjudgmental attitude and curiosity to your own sense of balance and coordination.

EXPLORATION 4.2
Mindful Movement

This practice is helpful in developing a greater awareness of your body's balance through slow, subtle movements.

- Stand with your feet slightly apart. See if you can stand perfectly still.
- Often there is a slight natural swaying of the body. Take a moment to notice that.
- Sense where your center of gravity is. Move sideways from left to right and front to back to help you find it.
- Exaggerate the sway of your body away from the center without losing your balance. Notice the points where the sway-out stops and the body starts returning to the center.
- Come back to the center and let your arms hang on each side of your body.

- Close your eyes and sense your arms' position. Rotate your shoulders, then your head; notice the sense of movement.
- Open your eyes and stand on one foot. Notice how your body adjusts its center of gravity. Note any falling or swaying.
- With both feet on the ground again, stretch or bend in any way you like, sensing the stretch, rotation, and sensations of your body. For example:
  - Stretch your arms as if reaching toward the sky.
  - Swing your arms from side to side.
  - Bend down and touch your toes.
  - Bend to the side.
  - Try yoga postures you know.

EXPLORATION 4.3
Mindful Walking (CD track 5; five minutes)

Walking meditation is a traditional mindfulness practice—indeed sitting and walking practice are often alternated during mindfulness meditation retreats. Here I describe a typical walking meditation that focuses on the sensations of moving your feet. You can do this meditation with your shoes on or do it in bare feet (being barefoot tends to make the sensations more pronounced).

- Stand with your feet together and eyes open.
- Slowly lift one of your legs and begin to walk.
- You can label the movement as "lifting and placing" or simply observe the movement without labeling.
- As you walk, notice the sensations of your feet touching the ground, especially the placement of the ball of the foot and the shift in weight felt there.

MINDFULNESS FOR ADHD

- If your mind wanders, gently bring your attention back to your feet. Remember that by returning to your intention, you are training your attention.
- At some point try taking one or two steps backward and notice how that feels.

Pointers on Mindful Walking

The traditional way of practicing walking meditation is to do it at a pace that is much slower than usual walking. This can at first feel unnatural or make you lose your balance. Simply notice whatever arises as you walk, but continue to do so, slowly. Alternatively, you can try it at your natural pace, or even at a fast pace. At this quicker pace, notice the movement of your entire leg or your arms instead of the sensations of your feet. As you walk, you can also gradually slow down and narrow your focus to your feet.

You can combine walking meditation with self-talk and imagination to strengthen the ability to move in other aspects of life. For example, you can imagine that moving the foot forward and placing it on the ground symbolizes being proactive and entering or starting something new. If you have a hard time starting tasks this may be a good practice for you.

Alternatively, instead of focusing on the ball of your foot moving forward, you can focus on the heel leaving the ground. You can imagine that lifting the heel of your foot symbolizes leaving things behind. If you have difficulties with transitions and letting go, this may be a good practice for you.

....

Mindfulness practice is inherently flexible and creative: As long as you're aware of what you're doing as you're doing it, you are practicing mindfulness.

....

Mind-Body Connection Is a Two-Way Street

Busy and overwhelmed, Mary developed a habitual tenseness. She had deep wrinkles between her eyebrows because she often pulled them together in a worried expression, even if there was nothing immediate to worry about. When she was out to dinner one night, her friend pointed it out to her. "Gosh, you look so tense and tired," her friend said.

That surprised Mary, as she was not fully aware of her expression. After the friend's comment, however, Mary resolved to check her facial expression throughout the day. When driving, at stoplights she would periodically check her face in her car visor's mirror. If it looked tense, she relaxed her forehead and her jaw. Quickly she noticed that the change in her face often prompted her to take a deep breath and channel relaxation to the rest of her body.

Our body and its facial expressions or posture often reflect how we feel on the inside. If we are sad, our face will reflect a downcast expression and our shoulders may droop. The whole body may project low energy and a feeling of dejection. We intuitively know this and often read others' emotions based on what their faces and their bodies communicate. But we may not always realize that this connection is *a two-way street*. Once we understand this, we can take advantage of the connection. We can shift and shape how we feel or think by purposely changing our facial expression or body posture.

For example, if a therapy patient wants to learn to speak up assertively, I often ask him or her to sit up straight before speaking. The change in posture often helps the person express his or her words with more empowerment than if they were sitting slumped on the couch. Shifting the body to get to a certain mind-body state is utilized in body-based psychotherapies, acting schools, and in sitting meditation. In meditation, correct body posture—usually upright and relaxed—is emphasized as a way to facilitate alertness as well as mental and emotional processing.

An interesting study led by Dr. Dana Carney at University of

Colombia demonstrated that changes in posture can have significant effects on the levels of power (testosterone) or stress (cortisol) hormones, behavior and inner feelings.[4] In this study, half of the participants were told to adopt a posture of high power and the other half a posture of low power. The postures of high power were what one could expect to see displayed by a high-level executive in a company meeting, including standing over the table with feet spread apart, stretching out in a chair with feet up on a table, keeping fingers interlaced behind the neck and elbows pointing outward. The postures of low power were what one could expect to see in a subservient and timid employee, including standing or sitting in a contracted and closed way, with arms close to the body as if "shrinking." The study showed that holding high-power postures for even one minute caused testosterone levels to rise, cortisol levels to drop, and increased inner feelings of being powerful and "in charge." Such participants were also more likely to take risk in a gambling task. Holding low-power poses produced the opposite effect.

Here are several methods for engaging your body to make a positive mind shift.

EXPLORATION 4.4
Shaking and Dancing Meditation

Shaking meditation is an example of active meditation. This practice comes from Kundalini yoga and often involves four sequential periods of shaking, dancing, standing or sitting still, and lying down. The periods are generally ten to fifteen minutes long, but here I present a shorter version modified from the one used by Dr. James Gordon of the Center for Mind-Body Medicine.[5] This exercise may seem silly at first, but be open to it and see how it feels. It can be a good way to release stress or restlessness as well as raise body energy. If you are a parent, try it with your kids for some extra fun!

PREPARE
- Create a CD or playlist to accompany you. It should have:
  - One to two minutes of initial silence so you can prepare for the meditation.
  - Five minutes of driving, rhythmic music that you can shake to.
  - Three to five minutes of music that makes you want to move and dance

START
- Place your feet shoulder-width apart and slightly bend your knees.
- Relax your shoulders and neck and take several deep breaths. Keep your eyes closed, or slightly open.

SHAKE
- When the music starts, begin shaking your whole body. Feel the energy moving up from your feet to your shoulders and your head.
- Practice letting go and allow yourself to *become* the shaking. Keep going, even if you're tired or bored, until this part of the music ends.
- When the music pauses, notice your breathing and physical sensations.

DANCE
- When the dancing music begins, let your body move as it wants to.
- Move freely and spontaneously. If you feel silly or embarrassed, notice that but keep moving.

STAND, SIT, OR LIE DOWN
- When the music stops, stand, sit, or lie down quietly.
- Notice your breathing and your body as you relax.

Other Ways to Take Advantage of the Mind-Body Connection

PRACTICE A "SOFT SMILE"

As you read this, move the corners of your mouth up into a small, gentle smile. If you chronically hold tension in your jaw, make sure there's some space between your upper and lower teeth, and then smile. Notice if there's a corresponding subtle shift in how you feel inside. Often there may be a corresponding "inner smile" or lightening feeling, since such smiling can signal relaxation to the rest of the body. Practice the soft smile (even if only for a few seconds) throughout your day—it may change your entire outlook.

DO AEROBIC EXERCISE

Any aerobic activity can shift your breathing and body energy, and improve your concentration, thinking, and mood. Whenever you're stuck on a task or problem, take a break to do something physically active. This could be going to the gym, taking a walk around the block, or simply doing some stretching or jumping jacks in your room. Then reengage with the task. You may notice increased motivation and new insights in dealing with the problem.

GET A MASSAGE (OR SIMILAR ACTIVITY FOR DEEP MUSCLE RELAXATION)

A massage can quickly make your body go from tense to very relaxed. If you haven't ever tried it, go get one (or get your friend or partner to give you one) and notice the shift in the state of your body and mind with enhanced awareness. Other activities that can help your muscles relax include yoga, taking a hot bath, or sitting in a sauna.

Can you think of other ways to access this state of relaxation?

There are different styles of learning, and many people prefer one over another. The main types are:

1. Visual (learning best by seeing)
2. Auditory (learning best through hearing)
3. Reading and writing (just what it sounds like)
4. Kinesthetic or tactile (learning best by doing)

Many children and adults with ADHD report having a preference for visual and kinesthetic learning. If that includes you, making information external and engaging your body in the learning process can be of great help. When studying a topic, make study aids that help you engage with the information through the body and that encourage using your hands. Write or draw the information out, make flash cards, or build models.

When learning a new life skill, use body movement, together with imagery, to instill the feeling or attitude. For example, if you need to be more assertive, imagine speaking assertively with the person you have difficulty with. Practice sitting or standing up straight and moving your arm in a decisive "no!" gesture. The movement can help you tap into the assertive energy in your body.

One the other hand, if you tend to automatically disagree with others in conversations (this is often a case for adults with ADHD and an oppositional/defiant trait) visualize speaking with another person with a stance of openness and without having to argue back. Reinforce the imagery by holding your palms in an open and receptive position.

Working with Difficult Body Sensations: Pain and Restlessness

ADHD adults often describe restlessness as a very uncomfortable, almost painful feeling that they desperately want to get rid of. Here we explore mindful ways of working with difficult body sensation such as actual physical pain or significant restlessness.

In mindfulness, it is often said that *pain is inevitable, but suffering is optional.*

That means that while we cannot always avoid pain (or discomfort, like restlessness in ADHD), we can limit the related suffering. Our attitude and relationship to the discomfort can make a huge difference in what we experience. For example, much ongoing suffering comes from one or more of the following:

- Having a negative reaction to the discomfort (dread, fear, anger)
- Resisting the discomfort or wanting things to be different (e.g., keeping busy all the time, looking for explanations at all cost even if there may not be one, blaming others)
- Overidentifying with the discomfort (e.g., *"my* pain" versus "the knee pain," or *"I am* restless" versus *"I notice* restlessness")
- Creating a story about the discomfort (e.g., "This will never end" or "I am powerless")

By accepting and investigating the discomfort in a nonreactive way, using mindfulness, suffering can be minimized. The following story illustrates how.

Mindfulness of Physical Pain

John woke up with a headache. Work had been stressful, and he had a lot of tension in his neck and shoulders. He was annoyed by the headache and took several over-the-counter pain medications to get rid of it. This dulled the pain, but a nagging discomfort remained throughout the day. John was increasingly irritated and impatient for it to go away. These feelings made his neck even tenser, which increased the pain. Frustrated, he called his friend Robert, a physician. Robert was in the midst of taking a mindfulness-based stress reduction class (MBSR), so he decided to try mindfulness with John. Here's how it went:

Robert: How about we use mindfulness to work with your pain?

John: OK, what do I do?

Robert: First, see if you can accept the pain—don't fight it. You don't have to like it—just don't push it away with impatience. Instead, become curious about it. See if you can explore the pain simply as a body sensation.

John: OK, well, my pain is bad...

Robert: See if you can describe it not as "my pain," but in a less personal way. Describe it more as a sensation, for example, "there's a sharp feeling" or "there's a throbbing sensation."

John: Well, it's a steady pressure around the forehead.

Robert: What are the boundaries? Is it the entire forehead, just part of it, or other areas, too?

John: It's mostly a stretch between my forehead and my temples.

Robert: Is it changing, or remaining the same?

John: It's kind of pulsing up and down.

Robert: What else is there?

John: Well, it's kind of worse now that I'm paying attention to it. I'm afraid it'll never go away!

Robert: That can happen sometimes. First notice the fearful thought as simply a thought, and then shift your attention to a comfortable spot like your breath or your palms. Focus there for a bit and relax.

John focused on his breath for a short while.

John: I do feel a little better.

Robert: OK, when you're ready, put your attention back on the painful area again and notice the sensations or your thoughts or feelings a bit more. When it starts to feel like too much, go back to your breath.

As Robert guided John through this mindfulness-of-pain approach, John noticed the headache lessening its hold. He felt more relaxed and the overall discomfort was reduced.

EXPLORATION 4.5
Working with Restlessness

In the example above, Robert demonstrated how to bring mindful attention to physical pain. Working with restlessness is much the the same. We can (1) put our attention on uncomfortable sensations with acceptance and curiosity, and (2) move our attention to a place that is neutral or more comfortable, like the breath, the palms, or sounds in the environment. This back-and-forth movement can help us to be with the discomfort in a new, healing way.

The next time you notice that you're feeling restless, try this approach:

- Get curious about the sensation of restlessness. See it as something you can investigate and observe with mindfulness.
- Notice different sensations and describe them in your mind. Use neutral terms (e.g., a buzzing energy, some tingling, the urge to move) versus "my" or "I am."
- As you explore this, are you aware of any thoughts or feelings present—for example, "I can't stand this"? Note these as phenomena you can watch without acting on them.
- After exploring the sensation of restlessness, turn to a neutral or safe focus, like your breath or sounds. Focus on the breath or sounds as long as you need. Then check in to the sensation of restlessness again, with curiosity.

Tips on Working with Restlessness

If the sensation of restlessness seems unbearable, you can bring an attitude of gentleness and compassion to yourself as you investigate the sensation. For example, remind yourself, "I know that restlessness can be unbearable because of my ADHD" or "My ADHD makes it difficult to sit in this meeting." You can also imagine breathing into and holding the restlessness with compassion.

Also, see if you can find opportunities to *release the restless feeling*. Practice these strategies with mindfulness, noticing how your body (and mind) feels during them. For example:

- Go for a short walk and note how your restlessness feels during and after.
- Doodle or do another mindful distraction (knowing that you're distracting yourself on purpose) and periodically check in with your body.
- Make small, discrete movements, like rotating your wrists or ankles. Again, note the feelings of restlessness during and after.

Finally, consider consulting with your doctor about using medications to control feelings of restlessness. Just as with physical pain, if restlessness is significant, medication for ADHD can help.

Suggested Reminders for Practice

Two useful reminders for this step are:

- Check in with the body
- STOP (Stop, Take a breath, Observe the body, Proceed)

Post these signs in your environment wherever you're likely to see them.

....

Step 4 at a Glance

Formal Practice

- Each day, do one of the following: a ten-minute (or more, if you need) body scan, walking meditation, or shaking and dancing meditation.

- Use the STOPing practice with an emphasis on noticing body sensations.
- Bring more awareness to instances of slow, regular, or fast movements in your life, such as stretching, yoga, or tai chi (slow); walking (regular); or dancing or running movements (fast).
- Shift your body and mind through wearing a gentle smile, exercising, getting a massage, and so forth, and notice the sensations.
- Practice using the body to reinforce learning.
- Notice difficult sensations like pain or restlessness with mindfulness.
- In daily life, notice your body posture as you sit, walk, or stand. Pay special attention to the moments of transitions from lying down to sitting, then to standing, and then to walking. See if you can first notice when the urge to move arises and how your body follows.
- Bring more awareness to your body movements during your regular exercise routine.
- To develop a greater sense of balance, challenge yourself to do activities that involve balancing, such as dancing, yoga, tai chi, mountain biking, rock climbing, snowboarding, or skateboarding. For example, rock climbing requires exquisite attention to the present moment, in the need for mindful placement of one's hands and feet and being constantly aware of shifting body balance. Be patient with yourself if learning these activities takes you longer than others.

STEP 5   Observe Your Mind

Mindfulness of Thoughts

"My mind is always busy," exclaimed Carolyn. "If you ask me about one thing, that makes me think of a million other things."

"I noticed," I thought to myself. Carolyn was in my office for an evaluation of possible ADHD, and it was a struggle to keep her focused. Many of my questions were met with long descriptions and too many details. Other times, she veered to another topic. She seemed to be insightful, and her answers were often interesting or humorous—but they didn't always address the question.

Along with a restless body, a busy or restless mind is common with ADHD. This can be a curse and a blessing. Having a restless mind can make it difficult to focus and follow through on one's tasks without getting sidetracked or lost in thought. On the other hand, having lots of thoughts and ideas can lead to making unusual and intriguing connections between things. Many adults with ADHD exhibit "out-of-the box" thinking and creativity due to their incessantly curious mind.

In this step of the program, we will learn to watch thinking with mindfulness. We'll focus on observing ADHD-mind patterns when it's fairly easy to do so—when there's no strong pull or emotional charge. (This step is a preparation for step 6, where we'll learn to observe and transform difficult thoughts and emotions.)

The ADHD Mind

In ADHD, thought flow is often irregular. Ideas can frequently branch out or jump from place to place. On the other hand, there may also be a tendency to get stuck in one way of thinking or to obsess about something—a kind of inflexible flow.

With frequent jumps in thinking, the content of ADHD mind may sometimes look like a disorganized closet and sometimes like a zigzaggy road that ultimately reaches a novel insight. Sometimes the content of the ADHD mind is out of balance or skewed. For example, the thinking may be overly optimistic or overly pessimistic (see below).

Self-Perception and ADHD

Accurate self-perception seems to be difficult in ADHD. For example, positively biased self-perceptions—reporting higher competence than what the actual performance shows—are common in ADHD children.[1] This kind of overestimation in children is found across the board in social, academic, and behavioral domains. It may be in part a result of certain cognitive deficits, and it may have a protective role in early years; however, its full impact is still unknown. (At the same time, children with ADHD are typically accurate in their perceptions of others' performance.[2])

The problem with accurate self-perception is also shown in adults with ADHD. In a 2005 study adults with ADHD self-reported higher competence as drivers than their observed performance and their driving record showed.[3] In contrast, a 2007 study among college-aged students, by contrast, suggested that ADHD students tended to underestimate their academic performance.[4]

In my clinical experience, many adults with ADHD, before even being introduced to mindfulness, are able to notice or joke about their mental process. Perhaps the repeated experience of living with an unruly, frustrating, and skewed mind makes it easier for them to see their thoughts as somewhat separate from themselves. However, despite this general knowledge, it can still be difficult for people with ADHD to notice the very moments when their mind jumps or gets stuck in unbalanced thinking.

Mindfulness of Thinking

The mindfulness-based approach to thinking is different from traditional psychotherapy in that it teaches us to experience a *different relationship* to our thoughts before attempting to focus on their content. Mindfulness first invites us *to watch or witness the flow of thinking*. Instead of being caught up in the narrative in our head, we are invited to observe our thinking as an ever-changing stream, similar to watching clouds float across the sky. This shift in perspective weakens the grip of unhelpful thinking. A 2007 study by Norman Farb at the University of Toronto showed that mindfulness training can weaken the tendency to be caught in an inner story and analysis of yourself[5] and promotes focus on direct experience. This is important since habitual self-analysis can make one more vulnerable to unhelpful rumination, anxiety, and depression.[6] In contrast, focus on present-moment experience, as in mindfulness, has been demonstrated to promote well-being.[7]

EXPLORATION 5.1
Mind Like a Sky (CD track 6; eight minutes)

- Sit comfortably and close your eyes. Become grounded in the present moment by noticing your breathing.

- When you feel settled, imagine a spacious blue sky with white clouds floating across it.
- Sense your awareness as being like the blue sky, vast and spacious, larger than the passing clouds. With such awareness, you can watch your thoughts and feelings as if they were clouds coming and going.
- As you watch them, label your thoughts and feelings without personalizing them—for example, "oh, there is worry," "sadness," "remembering."
- Notice that, just like clouds, your thoughts may go by quickly or slowly. They may be linked with each other or floating separately. They may appear light and fluffy or dark and heavy.
- As you watch your thoughts flow, see if you can sense *the space between them*. This space—the space of open awareness—is a place where you can observe your mind without being pulled by it. It is the space from which you can note thoughts and feelings but choose to not act on them.
- As you do this exercise, it is easy to get lost in thinking—to go into the clouds and become enveloped by the content of your thoughts and feelings. Whenever that happens, become aware of your breath and reground yourself in the present moment. Then return to watching your mind.

As a child, I used to love lying on the grass and watching clouds float across the sky. I remember being amazed at how the clouds moved and changed from moment to moment. Not knowing how they would configure themselves, I would simply wait to see what would evolve. Without realizing it then, I was experiencing open, receptive awareness.

Tips and Variations

Other images or metaphors can also be used to explore mindfulness of thoughts and feelings. For example, you can imagine yourself standing on the bank of a river and watching your thoughts and feelings as if they are leaves floating by in the water. Or you can imagine that you're at a movie theater watching your thoughts, memories, and feelings projected on a screen. Use the imagery that helps you get to an open and monitoring perspective, whatever helps you to become a witness to your thinking. Also, try the next exercises, "Watching Your Thinking under a Tree" or "Mind Like an Ocean," for alternative ways to connect with open awareness.

In general, thoughts can be challenging to observe because they can be subtle or, alternatively, they can be strong and difficult to step back from (especially worry, obsessive thinking, or self-critical thoughts). If you find yourself unable to simply witness your thoughts and feelings as described in this chapter, you can skip this step and move ahead to step 6 (Manage Your Emotions) before returning here. The tools described there can help you observe strong or difficult thoughts that typically have negative feelings attached to them.

EXPLORATION 5.2
Watching Your Thinking under a Tree

- Go to a park that has trees with many branches and leaves.
- Find a spot where you can lie down under such a tree, and look up at the complex network of leaves and branches above you.
- The network usually makes it hard to fixate on one point; if so, notice how your attention dances from one spot to another.
- However, if you find that you tend to fixate on one spot, see if you can allow your attention to relax and move

between the branches and leaves. This relaxed "dance of attention" can open up your awareness and make it easier to watch your thinking without being caught up in it.

- Notice what thoughts arise as you rest under the tree.
- After a while, close your eyes and see if you can continue to watch your thinking with the same spacious awareness.

EXPLORATION 5.3
Mind Like an Ocean

- Sit comfortably and close your eyes. Imagine that your mind is like a big blue ocean, vast and deep. And just like there are waves on the surface of the ocean, your thoughts can be restless, agitated, or choppy. Yet underneath there is always calm water, no matter how restless the ocean's surface gets. This is also the case with the human mind.
- Keeping the ocean in your mind, see if you can connect with this sense of deep calm within you: the space of stillness from which the restless thoughts, like ruffled waves, can be watched from a distance.
- As you imagine the ocean with its waves at the surface and deep calm beneath, see if you can remain aware of your breath or your body. Practice staying grounded in this awareness as you envision the ocean and watch your thinking.

Mindful Daydreaming

Both ADHD life experience and mindfulness practice give us plenty of opportunities to experience daydreaming. In steps 1–3, we focused on catching and interrupting the wandering mind by focusing our attention back to a present moment (for example, by returning our attention to the breath). Now, we explore daydreaming with awareness.

The Science of Daydreaming

Research by scientists including Dr. Jonathan Schooler at the University of California–Santa Barbara, and Dr. Kalina Christoff at the University of British Columbia suggests that one part of the mind is the locus for analytical thinking and a conscious sense that "I am thinking these thoughts." Another part of the mind is associated with spontaneous mind-wandering and daydreaming. Doing routine, automatic tasks often initiates this second, daydreaming, side of the mind.[8]

Many brain studies have shown that when the analytical side of the mind is active, the executive function network typically becomes active as well. By contrast, when a person is daydreaming, it's typical that the brain regions called the "default network" activate. The default network is often thought to be a reflection of how the brain operates during ostensibly idle, unproductive time. However, this pattern is not always so. A 2009 neuroimaging study by Dr. Christoff showed that there are times during daydreaming when the default network and the executive network are turned on simultaneously.[9] It's as if the daydreaming mind is working out a problem. On the brain level, such active daydreaming looks similar to times of creative thinking and problem-solving with insight.

Christoff's study also suggested that active daydreaming appeared to happen most often when the participants were completely unaware that they were daydreaming. However, a habit of purposeful checking-in with your mind may be the way to capitalize on such moments of creative thinking, suggests Dr. Schooler.[10] It seems that having periodic mindful awareness of just where your mind is and what it's doing can allow you to recognize potentially insightful thoughts. With such awareness, you also have a choice about whether to refocus on the task at hand or let your mind roam some more.

The hallmark of daydreaming is being completely lost in thought—unaware of what's going on around you and unaware that you have drifted away from what's happening in the present moment. However, it's possible to daydream *and know that we are daydreaming*. We can develop this ability for mindful daydreaming in several ways.

- When you have some free time, get comfortable and allow the mind to roam for a while. You can pick a topic (for example, ponder your last vacation) or simply let your thoughts generate content on their own. If you can, sit back and watch how your thoughts evolve. This takes some practice, and it may be easy to get lost in your thoughts. However, even if that happens, you can practice remembering the train of thought and writing it down afterward.
- If you spontaneously become aware that you've been daydreaming, see if you can trace your thoughts backward. Be curious about the course your mind took and what prompted you to shift out of daydreaming.
- Being engrossed in a movie is a lot like daydreaming. When watching a film, see if you can periodically acknowledge to yourself that you are engrossed in it.

Making Room for the "Aha!" Moment

Inventors and creative people have often come up with some of their greatest ideas when they were not actively trying to solve a problem—by having a sudden "aha" moment in the midst of doing something unrelated or mundane. Such examples—and now the brain studies, too—suggest that doing repetitive, familiar, or boring tasks can turn on the daydreaming, insightful mind. Thus we can make a point to do such activities on purpose in order to tap into our "aha!" moments. Here are some examples:

- When you're stuck on a problem, take a break. Do something repetitive like chopping vegetables, knitting, or folding the laundry. See if your mind revisits the problem on its own. Often a solution comes to mind when you let your mind roam freely.

- You can also watch waves, water in a stream, or fish in an aquarium. Anything that gets your mind to relax and roam.

- Outline a problem in your mind before you do a mindfulness meditation practice. Then let go of the effort to solve it, and focus on the meditation. As you do so, you'll let go of the analytical mind and also, at times, slip into daydreaming. See if an insight comes to you during or after the meditation.

A Famous "Aha!" Moment

The Greek mathematician and physicist Archimedes is said to have figured out how to measure the volume of an irregular object while he was taking a bath. The realization of the principle of displacement came to him when he observed that the level of water in the tub rose as he got in. The traditional story tells us that Archimedes got so excited about the sudden insight that he ran out of the tub naked into the streets, yelling, "Eureka!" ("I've found it!")

Mindfulness of Unhelpful Thinking

Joe, a teacher in his fifties, reflected on his experience with mindfulness: "Before I learned mindfulness," he said, "I didn't really understand what it meant to 'be living in the dream of the mind.'...I understood being caught in thinking or daydreaming but didn't realize you can go through life thinking you're awake and aware, yet have an 'old film' going on in your mind. Through mindfulness, and my work in psychotherapy, I came to understand that we are often conditioned to see things in a certain way or to react in a certain way without full awareness. With mindfulness, I can watch my old patterns....I now accept that they can come up—they are part of my past. But I can choose to unhook myself from them. I can also choose to bring on more helpful thinking—the thinking that comes from the wise part of myself."

Mindfulness practice gives us an opportunity to experience a space between us and our thinking. Such moments can be freeing. Moreover, in those moments we can connect with the part of ourselves that is wise and can guide us to a more positive outcome. This wise self can recognize what is happening with clarity, help us fully accept it, and decide what should be changed. This tension between acceptance and change is a key theme in mindfulness-based approaches such as Dialectical Behavioral Therapy (DBT), a therapy developed by psychologist Dr. Marsha Linnehan to help patients with suicidal thinking and impulsivity.[11] This approach also has been successfully adapted for ADHD adults, as they often struggle with intense negative reactions and unbalanced thinking.[12]

Balancing of Acceptance and Change

Mindfulness training, spiritual traditions, and therapies that draw from them emphasize that the courageous acceptance of what is—sometimes called radical acceptance—is required for effective change and healing to happen. This sentiment is also expressed in the widely known Serenity Prayer[13] often used by Alcoholics Anonymous and other 12-Step programs.

> God, grant me the serenity
> To accept the things I cannot change,
> Courage to change the things I can,
> And wisdom to know the difference

Judgmental Thinking

Judgmental, hypercritical, or disapproving thinking is often automatic and can be a barrier to being open and receptive to experiences. It also creates a barrier to having a compassionate relationship with yourself and others. Judgmental thoughts about oneself (negative self-talk) and self-doubt are often reported by adults with ADHD. These adults typically have grown up hearing critical comments about their performance, like "You haven't gotten your homework done yet? Stop being lazy and get to it!"

Such messages often get internalized with age, forming an "inner critic." This negative thinking can lead some to create a story about themselves that starts out with "I can't," "I'm dumb," or "Something's wrong with me." Many adults with ADHD carry such stories within themselves and may not realize how much this negative self-talk can hold them back in life.

Sometimes I readily hear the inner critic in what a person with ADHD says, but other times it's covered over by a happy or confident demeanor. Underneath, however, there still may be feelings of insecurity and negative self-talk. Mindfulness can help us notice and understand the full extent of our self-judgment. Let's look at how to do this in more detail.

OBSERVING JUDGMENTAL THOUGHTS

Become curious about judgmental thoughts that come up for you in the course of your day. They may be directed at yourself or people around you. As a mindful exercise, try counting your judgmental thoughts in the course of one day—you may be surprised at what you find.

Counting Judgmental Thoughts

As part of her at-home mindfulness practice, Mina, a young college student, counted her judging thoughts during one day. "I started paying attention to how quickly negative judgments came up whenever I interacted with others," she said. "When my professor handed me my test with a C on it, I thought, 'She is such a bitch.' Looking at my grade I later caught myself thinking, 'I am such a failure.' As I continued to observe, when talking with another student, I caught myself thinking, 'What a ditz.' It was a revelation to me how much such thoughts came up. I counted at least a hundred of them in one day."

As you observe judgmental thoughts, you may actually notice *judgmental thoughts about having judgmental thoughts,* such as, "I am so awful for having all these negative judgments!" That's OK—just notice it as another judgmental thought.

NEUTRALIZING STRONG AND PAINFUL SELF-JUDGMENTAL THOUGHTS

Sometimes harsh self-judgments cause us pain or shame. Mindfulness provides some ways to neutralize such thinking and regain a balanced perspective. For example, you can remind yourself that the thoughts, even if they feel true, are *just thoughts* after all. To further help you step back from them, shift your attention to your body and notice your breath and other body sensations. You may become aware of an emotion that's fueling the negative thinking. See if you can have an attitude of self-compassion at that moment. If the negative thoughts and emotion are intense, use the tools described in step 6 (Manage Your Emotions).

Being Too Hard on Yourself—Julie's Story

Julie, one of my adult ADHD patients, was describing to me a mistake she'd made at work. She was discussing her project with her boss and a couple of coworkers, but she couldn't remember her main client's name. She had a momentary mental block—a fairly common occurrence in ADHD—and she called the client's company by a different name. She felt embarrassed and humiliated in front of her coworkers. "I am so, so stupid!" she said to me, with tears in her eyes. "My brain is like a sieve, it just doesn't hold anything! They must think I'm an idiot."

I encouraged Julie to have compassion for herself about making mistakes. While initially she found it hard to do so—I had to help her to accept her work mistake as part of her ADHD difficulties—with time she was able to have more self-compassion on her own.

DEVELOPING COMPASSIONATE AND SUPPORTIVE THINKING

If you were sitting across from your friend who was struggling, what would you say? Often we are kinder and more supportive toward others than we are toward ourselves. So whenever your inner critical voice rears its head, see if another part of you can offer the advice you would give your friend in a similar situation. Such a supportive self-coaching voice is nicely described in the following story, paraphrased from a cognitive-behavioral-therapy workbook for adults with ADHD:[14]

Coach A versus Coach B

Johnny is a little boy practicing baseball. He's standing in the outfield, ready to catch a fly ball, but he misses it despite his efforts. Coach A runs up to him and starts yelling: "I can't believe you missed that ball! You can't do anything right! You better shape up for next time or you'll be sitting on the bench!"

How do you think Johnny feels now? Probably he's less confident, tense, and about to cry. His chances of catching the ball next time are not much better—if anything, they're worse, as he's now affected by Coach A's negative words. He may be discouraged from playing baseball ever again, or no longer enjoy the game.

Now, let's replay the same scene with Coach B. Johnny is practicing catching baseballs and misses a fly ball. Coach B comes to the scene and says: "Well, you missed that one. Here's what I want you to remember: fly balls always look like they're farther away than they really are. How about you take a few steps backward and run forward if you need to? Let's see how you do next time."

How do you think Johnny feels now? Probably he's more confi-

dent, as he received some constructive and supportive feedback. His chance of doing better is higher, he's motivated to keep trying, and he's more likely to enjoy the game.

Notice that Coach B did not say, "You did great!" or "It's no big deal, just keep practicing." While these kinds of comments may be helpful for some, they also may be a disservice to the boy, who is struggling and does not know how to proceed. It's the authentic and kind approach—with specific feedback—that really makes a difference.

Keeping this story in mind, if you notice your own thoughts sounding more like "Coach A," see if you can bring on "Coach B" instead.

ADHD Mind Traps

In addition to judgmental thinking, some thoughts are a sort of mind trap: they get you stuck. In ADHD, these mind traps often come from thinking that is *polarized:* where things are extreme in either a positive or negative direction. With mindfulness you can notice when such thinking, also known as cognitive distortions,[15] arises and then choose to rebalance it. (If the thinking creates a lot of problems in your life, tools from cognitive-behavioral therapy (CBT) can further help you change such thinking.) Here are some examples of polarized thinking:

All-or-none thinking: Seeing yourself, others, or situations as all good or all bad, or seeing only one way of doing something. For example: "I have to be right all the time," or "I have to get all of this done today," or "I will never get it done," "This all sucks," "This will never end," and so forth. Words like "never" or "always" are cues that this kind of thinking is occurring.

Blaming others or blaming oneself: Blaming others is frequent in oppositional-defiant disorder, which is diagnosed in up to 50 percent of children with ADHD. When such children grow up, the blaming habit can continue, which leads to anger and frustration in relationships.

The polar opposite of habitually blaming others is habitually blaming yourself. For example, "I must have done something to cause this." You tend to over-personalize events and automatically hold yourself responsible when something goes wrong. In this thinking, you tend to overlook others' contributions to the problem and continuously erode your self-esteem.

Magnifying or minimizing: In magnifying, you tend to overestimate—or blow out of proportion—an aspect of a situation or the consequences of a problem. Catastrophizing, or imagining a worst-case scenario, is an example of magnifying. For example: "This mistake means I'll be fired." When stuck in this mind trap, you tend to discount positive information like "It's just a small mistake," and instead think "This mistake is horrible."

Conversely, when minimizing, you tend to shrink or overlook facts about others, yourself, or situations. For example, you may discount your own abilities and talents or overlook others' faults. This kind of thinking may also contribute to minimizing a consequence for an action or being unrealistic about your limitations. It can be a sort of wishful thinking, for example: "I can stay an extra hour and still make it to the airport." Difficulties with mapping out steps involved in a task and underestimating how long they take—an executive function impairment—can contribute to this problem in ADHD.

Making assumptions or not seeing the obvious: You convince yourself you know what others are thinking and feeling, based on conjecture. You think you know what's going on even if there's no direct evidence. For example, you assume your friend is mad at you because she didn't call you back. The assumptions are often negative, but positive assumptions can also create problems. For example, you may assume that because your boss didn't mention the regular weekly meeting in his last e-mail, you are free to do something else. You don't verify the assumption with your colleagues, and you fail to show up at the required meeting.

The opposite of making assumptions is having all the evidence in front of you yet being unable to draw a proper conclusion. In ADHD, this can happen as a result of problems with making transitions, executive function difficulties, or being colored by emotions. For example, you have a doctor's appointment at 5 p.m. and plan to leave your house at 4 p.m. so you can stop by a store on the way. You don't leave your house until 4:45 p.m., and even though it's now too late to go to the store, you proceed with the original plan.

Rigid, rules-based thinking versus lack of rules: This mind trap involves words like "should" or "have to," as in, "It has to be done like this," or "I shouldn't have to do this." The rules can be overly rigid and unrealistic and set you up for feeling guilty or depressed if you don't meet your own standards. For example, if you think, "I have to get this done today" and then you fail to do so, you may get discouraged and not try the next day. Having rigid standards for yourself can also make you resentful if others break the rules.

The opposite, "I don't have to," means that you don't have enough rules for yourself or tend to break them too often. This can derail the development of self-discipline and self-motivation needed to achieve goals.

To rebalance polarized thinking, remember that reality is more often gray than black-and-white. As a self-check, when you feel stuck or upset, ask yourself:

- Is my thinking balanced right now?
- Am I stuck in one of the mind traps? If so, which one?
- Is there another way of looking at this?

Suggested Reminders for Practice

- Post an image of the sky and clouds in your environment, as a reminder to become a witness of thoughts and feelings.
- Use the STOPing practice to observe thoughts. Create a reminder sign that says:

  S = Stop

  T = Take a breath

  O = Observe your thoughts

  P = Proceed

- Remind yourself to be Coach B (balanced) rather than Coach A (angry). Post a reminder:

  Coach B, Not Coach A

- Use an image of an ocean wave as a reminder of the calm that lies below thoughts and feelings.

....

Step 5 at a Glance

Formal Practice

- Do ten minutes (or more) of open-awareness sitting meditation each day. Use sky or ocean imagery if that is helpful to you, or simply practice witnessing your thinking stream.

Mindful Awareness in Daily Life

- If your mind feels scattered—or you notice yourself doing things in scattered way—let that be a reminder to take a deep breath, listen to the sounds around you, or check in to your body. Then imagine that you're stepping outside of the clouds and seeing them from some distance.

- Continue STOPing with enhanced open awareness of thinking. Observe any judgmental, critical, or polarized thoughts. Practice accepting them as well as changing them to nonjudgmental and balanced thoughts.
- Try journaling, especially so-called flow writing, in which the writing happens fast and without you censoring what flows out.
- Practice mindfulness of thinking and daydreaming.
- Make room for the "aha!" moment—stop solving a problem, take a break, and do something else relaxing or repetitive.

STEP 6   Manage Your Emotions

Mindfulness of Feelings

Jerry was establishing his own web and graphic design business. His friend Sarah asked him for help in designing a marketing brochure, and Jerry jumped on the opportunity. He worked very hard and gave Sarah a great deal on the price. She seemed pleased and told Jerry she would give him the next job. A couple of months later, however, Jerry learned that Sarah had a new brochure, designed by someone else. Jerry felt betrayed and angry. He immediately went to Sarah's office and told her that she wasn't a good friend. Sarah was surprised by the angry outburst and told Jerry that the other designer was an art student who did her brochure as a small school project. In terms of working with Jerry, Sarah was planning to have him re-do her web-site. Jerry felt embarrassed for overreacting and left the office, beating himself up for being a "hothead."

Like Jerry, many adults with ADHD have problems control-ling emotional reactions such as anger and frustration, which can lead to problems at work or with intimate relationships. These problems with *regulating emotions*—not only inattention or hyperactivity—are now being recognized as a very impor-tant, previously overlooked part of ADHD. In this step, we focus on acceptance and awareness of emotions, and we discuss mindfulness tools to manage them.

Emotions in ADHD

Emotions in ADHD were not studied much in the past, but that has been changing. A 2010 study by Dr. Russell Barkley and colleagues at the University of Oregon measured *emotional impulsiveness* in adults with ADHD and compared them to other patients at the same mental health clinic as well as to adults in the outside community.[1] The majority of participants with ADHD (up to 86 percent) reported one or more of the following:

- Chronic impatience
- Being quick to anger
- Being easily frustrated
- Overreacting
- Being easily excited
- Losing their temper
- Being touchy or easily annoyed

These emotional difficulties were almost as common as the traditional ADHD symptoms of inattention—and were more common than the symptoms of ADHD hyperactivity and impulsivity. They were also found to cause significant difficulties at work or school, a tendency for poor driving and a criminal record, lower marital satisfaction, and parenting stress.

While most of the listed impulsive emotions are negative, one of them, being easily excited or enthusiastic, may be considered positive in some contexts. However, in ADHD a quick, unchecked enthusiasm can lead you to taking on new projects when you're already very busy, forgetting your prior intention, or abandoning an established plan.

For example, you may plan to do some important errands, but upon running into a friend you excitedly decide to join him on a trip to a park. You may also disregard limitations (of time, health, or money): perhaps you don't consider the risks involved before saying yes to a new business venture, or you agree to go to a concert when you really should stay home and recuperate from a cold. Such excitement-driven decisions can lead to increased personal stress, as well as arguments and tension in relationships.

In my clinical work I often hear ADHD adults report other emotional difficulties in addition to emotional impulsiveness. Many complain of being insecure and self-doubting. Some can be easily excited but also easily discouraged. Many are sensitive to criticism and can experience shame over their shortcomings. Their emotional sensitivity often coexists with deficient emotional regulation skills—a sort of double whammy that can lead to frequent overreacting.

Clearly, managing emotions is a challenge for many adults with ADHD. They can have difficulties with recognition, regulation, and expression of emotions. Mindfulness can help with each of these aspects. The expression of emotions can be facilitated by mindful communication, which we'll discuss in step 7. But in this current step, we'll focus on internally recognizing and regulating emotional responses. We start by examining emotions in everyday life in a nonjudgmental way.

Emotions 101

Emotions are part of a being human, and they give meaning to our lives. They're evoked when we celebrate something as well as when we mourn our losses. Apart from frank mood disorders (feeling stuck in certain emotional states), emotions in and of themselves are neither good nor bad. Both positive and negative emotions are a natural and important part of life, and they serve as signals from our mind and body—signals that need to be understood and responded to skillfully. The key to emotional well-being is in how we *understand and relate to our emotions*—not whether we have them or what they are.

Here are four essential principles or insights into our emotions:

1. There are many shades of (and words for) emotions.

To better understand emotions, scientists have tried to categorize them. Most agree there are universal, basic emotions (anger, disgust, fear, joy, sadness, and surprise) as well as complex or mixed emotions (love, pride, embarrassment). Having words to describe our own emotions is important for successful emotional regulation. The table at the end of this step provides a list of words for labeling emotional states as you ponder them.

2. Emotions are a dynamic process and have a "refractory period."

Emotions are not static. They are "energy in motion" or "E-motion." Some compare emotions to comets—mobile balls of energy with tails trailing behind them. With our emotions there is often a sense of initial fiery intensity, an energy coursing through the body, and then there's often a residual effect (the tail of the comet). The latter is often called an emotion's *refractory period,* a time when our thinking, our inner state, and our actions are still colored by the emotion, even if the acute feeling has already subsided.[2] During this period we still may think and act differently from our usual manner, for example, being more jumpy after hearing a scary noise. We are not always fully aware of the refractory period and its effect on us, but with mindfulness we can more fully tune in to the effects and observe it rather than being driven by it.

3. Emotions arise in the mind and body.

An emotional reaction typically has three parts:

1. A feeling (for example, a sense of anger)
2. Body sensations (a tense back and clenched teeth)
3. Associated thoughts ("I hate this." "I want to hit you.")

4. Emotional reactions—their triggers, components, and related actions—can be broken down into a series of steps and stages, which we can learn to observe with enhanced awareness.

TRIGGER → EMOTIONS → AN URGE TO ACT → ACTION

An emotional reaction can happen quickly and without our full awareness, often driving us to an impulsive action. The ability to step back and watch emotional reactions *without necessarily acting on them* is key to emotional control. With practice, a mindful observation of emotion helps us recognize these triggers and urges and make a choice about what actions (if any) we want to take.

EXPLORATION 6.1
Pleasant, Unpleasant, and Neutral Events

For the next few days, bring curiosity to your emotional reactions. Create a table to record daily events and note how such events, even small ones, can evoke an emotional response: either positive, negative, or neutral.[3] You can watch your experiences as they're happening, or you can recall them later in the day. Using the following table as a guideline, as well as you can describe each part of the reaction (for instance, body sensations, feelings, and thoughts).

Day	Event / Trigger	Pleasant? Unpleasant? Neutral?	Body Sensations	Feelings	Thoughts	Actions (if any)
Mon	Lost my keys, again!	Unpleasant	– Tension in my neck and back – Heart racing – Sinking feeling in the stomach	– Anger at myself – Anxiety – Panic – Helplessness – Embarrassed	– I can't believe I did it again – I am such a loser – I don't have time to deal with this – I can't tell my husband	– Call a friend
	Watched a movie	Pleasant	– Relaxed body	– Interested – Amused	– It's been a while since I've seen a movie	– Sign up for Netflix

You can download a printable version of this table from www.shambhala.com/MindfulnessPrescription.

Day	Event / Trigger	Pleasant? Unpleasant? Neutral?	Body Sensations	Feelings	Thoughts	Actions (if any)
Tue						
Wed						
Thur						

Day	Event / Trigger	Pleasant? Unpleasant? Neutral?	Body Sensations	Feelings	Thoughts	Actions (if any)
Fri						
Sat						
Sun						

Mindfulness of Difficult Emotions

Difficulties with emotions often start with not having true acceptance: not accepting a situation, not accepting something about ourselves, or rejecting an underlying feeling. For example, not accepting that you have ADHD or habitually pushing away an angry feeling when in fact you are upset. In psychotherapy circles, this is called "experiential avoidance"—a tendency to avoid unpleasant feelings and thoughts, which creates secondary problems with worry, panic, anger, depression, addictions, or emotional numbing.

Mindfulness helps with acceptance, because it encourages us to notice with a nonjudgmental attitude simply what *is*—whether we like it or not. It allows us to take a courageous look at reality, without pushing away or clinging to anything and with the knowledge that something useful can be learned from each experience.

Witnessing Anxiety

Cheryl, a woman with ADHD, struggles with chronic fear and anxiety. At one of our meetings I encouraged her to listen to guided mindfulness meditations as a way of learning to observe and tolerate her anxiety. Two phrases really stuck with her: "Make space for this feeling" and "Use it." These became reminders for her to notice the anxiety without being overwhelmed by it. She also started accept the anxiety as a learning experience, acknowledging more deeply what it was telling her about herself or the situation at hand.

EXPLORATION 6.2
RAIN (CD track 7; seven minutes)

We've learned that we can observe everyday thoughts and feelings mindfully, like watching clouds in the sky. However, there are times when this isn't so easy. Difficult emotions can be like dark rain clouds or a hurricane: menacing harbingers of flooding. The RAIN practice can help you experience difficult feelings in a balanced way: so that even as you get wet, you do not drown.

In RAIN practice, each letter reminds us how to do a mindful observation:

R = Recognize

A = Accept

I = Investigate

N = Non-identify

The RAIN practice on the CD will have you use a memory of a recent upsetting event to explore each step. Later on, you can use this practice at the moment something provokes a strong feeling in daily life or when a strong feeling emerges during a quiet meditation.

- Sit in an upright position and relax by taking a few deep breaths. Keep your eyes closed or slightly opened.
- Bring to mind a difficult situation you may be experiencing right now, or think about a recent, upsetting event. Remember what was said or what exactly happened that upset you.
- Beginning with the letter *R, recognize* and label whatever feelings you notice, for example: "sadness," "anger," "hurt," or "embarrassment." Or maybe there's simply a feeling of numbness or disconnection. Simply be curious.

- Continue with the letter *A, accepting* what you notice. You don't have to like it—just accept the reality of your experience. Observe it without criticizing yourself for having or *not* having a particular reaction. Welcome the experience as a new insight.
- Next, with the letter *I, investigate* your experience a little more. Drop your attention into the body and notice any sensations present there: maybe some tensing up in the chest, clenching in the stomach, or a sinking feeling. Learn about your feelings from your body. As you investigate, do you notice any additional thoughts or reactions? Maybe a reaction to the difficult emotion, or a feeling of anger or shame for having the emotion? Keep recognizing and accepting all that is happening.
- As you do this, be kind and gentle with yourself—if at any point this exercise feels too difficult or painful, shift your attention to the breath or another comfortable or neutral spot. Return to the difficult place only if and when you feel ready to do so.
- Finally, like the letter *N* in RAIN, practice *not identifying* with the difficult experience. After all, it is merely a set of reactions and sensations: you are not defined by it. Simply watch your experience and learn from being with it.
- As you end, bring an attitude of appreciation to yourself for having the courage to be with the difficult experience. Know that even if an emotion or thought can feel strong or true, it does not need to have a hold on you. *You* can hold it with mindfulness.

Further Notes about the RAIN Practice

While RAIN is often used with negative feelings, you can do the steps with any feeling. Try it with a feeling of sudden excitement.

R = Recognize that you are having a flash of excitement

A = Accept that you are excited, and if it is impulsive, accept that.

I = Investigate the feeling in your body. Notice any urges or thoughts present. Perhaps there is a feeling of rush or sensations of tingling in your body.

N = Non-identify with the feeling; see the excitement as something you can observe without immediately acting on

When the feelings are particularly strong and difficult, you can incorporate writing down (or drawing) your thoughts and feelings. Such expression can help you step aside and make the experience less personal.

Q: Sometimes when I'm practicing mindfulness I'm told to "briefly note the thought or feeling and then return to the breath." Other times, like in the RAIN practice, I'm told to focus on the feeling and "investigate" it mindfully. How do I know when to do what?

This can be confusing when you first learn mindfulness. In the initial practices (steps 1–3) we often set an intention to be aware of one thing—for example, the breath. When distractions, thoughts, worries, feelings, or images come up and take our attention away, the instruction is to briefly note or label the distraction and then come back to the breath. You notice the thought or the feeling, but you don't engage with it and instead return to the intended anchor. Such practice helps to train focus, and helps loosen the grip of the busy or agitated mind. Any time you want to lessen the power of a feeling and feel calmer, use the practices in steps 1–3 (tuning to five senses or being with the breath, the body, or sounds).

However, there are times when the thoughts or feelings are persistent. For example, you sit down to do a meditation practice and keep coming back to your breath, but the feeling continues to be strong. Or in your daily life, you try to focus on your work, yet a feeling keeps bothering you. In those cases, it helps to turn your full attention to the distraction and investigate it a little more. Here you can use the RAIN practice. It's as if you decided to look it squarely in the eye. You may learn a lot from being with such a persistent guest.

Think of this analogy: Imagine relaxing with a newspaper at breakfast and suddenly you notice a tug on your pant leg or skirt. It's a young child wanting your attention. You may make a gesture to make the child go away because you want to continue reading. That may work for a while, but soon you feel another tug, then again, and again. If so, the wise thing is to stop reading and place your full attention on the child. Acknowledge him or her fully. See what the child wants. Sometimes this full acknowledgment satisfies them, and sometimes they also have an important message for you.

Responding to Our Emotions

In addition to acceptance of difficult emotions, mindfulness also forms a basis for skillfully managing emotions. Simply observing an emotional reaction with mindfulness, for example, can by itself create a positive emotional shift. We create a mental space—a space that allows us to decide what we want to do next in that moment. Consider the following example.

Jerry has always had a hot temper. In the past, his temper made him walk out on his job and it put a strain on his marriage. His wife, Ellen, often complained that when he got angry he would quickly "go from zero to a hundred." When angry, Jerry would lose himself in the reaction, raising his voice and cursing, no matter where he was. One time when they were eating dinner in a restaurant, a server was somewhat slow to respond and Jerry confronted him with cursing. The exchange made Ellen feel embarrassed and uncomfortable. Afterward Jerry would regret losing his cool and apologize to Ellen for his angry outburst, but episodes like this were hurting their relationship. Jerry agreed to take a mindfulness class to help him regulate his emotions. Halfway through the course he shared with the group that for the first time, he had a moment of catching himself and asking, "Why am I swearing?" This was the first time he had a glimpse of his excessive reaction without being fully engrossed and driven by it.

The space created by mindfulness gives us a chance to ask ourselves the following questions:

- Do I want to stay with the feeling, or do something to diminish it?
- Do I ignore the feeling (or the person that provoked it)?
- Do I respond?
- If I respond, when and how do I do it?

Mindful responses to emotion can include loving-kindness practice and attitudes of self-compassion, patience, and willingness. Let's look at these responses more closely in formal practice and as they can be used in daily life.

EXPLORATION 6.3
Loving-Kindness Meditation (CD track 8; seven minutes)

At times, ADHD causes much emotional pain, shame, despair, and hopelessness. Loving-kindness meditation helps transform these difficult feelings and creates a more caring and supportive attitude toward yourself. In this practice you send wishes of well-being to yourself and others. At the beginning, it's also a good practice to notice the relationship you currently have with yourself, by asking: is it hard or easy for me to do this practice?

- Settle into a comfortable sitting position. Take a couple of deep breaths and relax your body.

- In this practice, you are invited to cultivate positive emotions such as friendliness, love, kindness, and compassion for yourself and others. This isn't always easy, and it can feel a bit unnatural at first. Simply be open to what happens to you during this practice, noticing your experience from moment to moment.
- Bring to your mind a person in your life who easily evokes feelings of love and warmth: maybe a child, your significant other, or even a pet. Imagine them standing in front of you.
- Notice how you feel as you bring them to mind. There may be a feeling of happiness or warmth in your body, a smile on your face, or a sense of an open heart. This feeling is loving-kindness—a feeling of caring and friendliness.
- As you imagine your loved one, see if you can silently wish him or her happiness and well-being. You can use words such as "May you be happy, may you be safe, may you be healthy and live with ease." Or come up with your own phrases reflecting love and kindness.
- Gently repeat the wishes of well-being several times. As you do, continue to notice how your body feels.
- If at any point you find that your attention has wandered off, gently bring it back and begin again.
- Now see if you can extend the wishes of loving-kindness to yourself. You may repeat words like "May I be happy, may I be safe, may I be healthy and live with ease. May I accept myself as I am." Or use your own words.
- Notice how it feels to extend caring wishes to yourself. If you notice that you're not feeling anything, or that you're feeling something else other than loving-kindness, just bring curiosity to that. Notice what's arising in your thoughts and in your body. You can learn from this experience, no matter what it's like.
- Traditionally, loving-kindness is extended in stages, starting with oneself and extending to those we love, those

we feel neutral about, those we consider our enemies, and then all beings.

- See if you can send out loving-kindness to other people in your life. Imagine opening your heart and extending loving-kindness in all directions: to people you care about, people whom you feel neutral about or don't know, people who are suffering. Touch them with thoughts such as "May we all be happy; may we all be safe, healthy, and live with ease; may we all be compassionate and gentle with ourselves and others; may we all experience joy and well-being."
- See if you can extend loving-kindness to people you find difficult or who have harmed you in some way. See what comes up for you and observe whether you're ready to send such wishes.

··

May we all be happy; may we all be safe, healthy, and live with ease; may we all be compassionate and gentle with ourselves and others; may we all experience joy and well-being.

··

Notes on Loving-Kindness Practice

If it is hard for you to keep in mind the given phrases of loving-kindness, come up with your own phrases that are easy for you to remember. They can be as short as "May you be happy and well." In this meditation, you can also use an image instead of words, for example, imagining the loving-kindness to be a warming light coming out of your heart and touching others.

If it's difficult for you to connect with a feeling of care and kindness for yourself, find a picture of yourself as a child and practice offering the wishes of love and kindness to that child. Notice how it feels to you to do this practice in this way.

Some people need the help of an another person to connect with kind feelings toward themselves. Having a caring friend, spouse, or therapist can help. Try imagining the person who cares about you sending you good wishes. (If you're a spiritual person, it can be helpful to think of God, a Higher Power, or the Universe and the love you receive from that source during this meditation.)

Bear in mind that it's difficult to send loving-kindness to people who have hurt you in some way. You may first have to allow yourself to experience the anger and grief the person has caused. When you feel ready, practice loving-kindness for them, even if it's difficult. Such practice often frees your heart from negative feelings.

Q: Sometimes all I can do is recognize that I am having a really hard time emotionally. I'm feeling bad, and it's too hard for me to breathe through it or investigate my feelings. I want to feel better right then and there. What can I do?

There are times when negative feelings can be very intense. Dialectical Behavioral Therapy offers useful strategies (so-called distress-tolerance skills)[4] that can bring relief from the intensity. Here are some tools from DBT for doing that:

- *Distracting yourself.* Do enjoyable activities; push the distressing situation out of your mind by getting busy with something else (for instance, helping others) or doing something with a strong sensation (like taking a cold shower, eating spicy food, or smelling an intense scent).
- *Taking care of your physical health.* For example, make sure that if you are physically suffering you get the proper treatment; make sure you eat properly, you get enough

sleep, you exercise, and you avoid excessive drugs and alcohol that can make your emotions extreme.

- *Doing something that comforts or relaxes you.* For example, you can call your spouse or your friend, spend time with your pet, use soothing imagery, read an encouraging book, pray, write in a journal, or take a vacation.

The Power of Compassion, Patience, Forgiveness, and Willingness

In daily life, a conscious decision to have compassion, patience, and forgiveness for yourself or others can transform moments of strong negative feelings. Here are some examples.

Self-Compassion

Barb is an accomplished educator who also has ADHD. She was asked to give an interview for an online magazine, which was to be recorded and then transcribed. Before the interview, Barb felt nervous and doubtful that she could perform well. Nevertheless, she accepted the journalist's phone call and did the best she could answering his questions.

A couple of weeks later, the transcript of the interview was posted online. As Barb read it, she immediately felt mortified and embarrassed: the transcript showed how she tended to jump from one topic to another. Some of her answers started to address the initial questions but then veered off to talk about some other, unrelated, topic. The journalist had to re-ask the question on a couple of occasions. The transcript also included run-on sentences and repetitions. Barb stopped reading and had to close her laptop. She felt exposed and stupid.

Feeling agitated and sick to her stomach, she started pacing in her living room. "What will my students think if they see this?" she thought. She was starting to get angry at herself for being so inept. But then she also remembered to practice self-compassion during such moments. In her mind, she asked, "Can I be compassionate to myself right now? Can I be compassionate about how my ADHD mind works?"

She felt a shift; the shame and the anger at herself lessened, and her tense muscles softened. She also did few minutes of a brief loving-kindness practice, repeating in her mind, "May I be OK, may I accept myself just as I am," several times while focusing on her breathing. This neutralized the intense negative feelings and helped her step back from the situation. She wasn't happy about how the interview turned out, but she no longer beat herself up about it. She was able to return to it later and read the whole thing without the intense negative reaction. She could appreciate that the interview still had some useful information for others, despite the ADHD-style disorganization apparent in her answers.

Self-compassion versus self-esteem: Studies show that having self-compassion is more important than having high self-esteem. Self-compassion not only buffers us against negative feelings in daily life, but it's been shown also to help people *acknowledge their role in negative events* without feeling overwhelmed with negative emotion.[5]

Patience

Jeff, an adult with ADHD, would frequently get stressed and frustrated when getting his eleven-year-old son, Patrick, ready for school. Patrick also has ADHD, and he can be difficult to get out the door. He's often sluggish, his school things are typically all over the place, and he generally doesn't know where his shoes and coat are. Having a system of getting ready the night before has helped, but Patrick can still be disorganized in the morning, making his father wait with him. However, Jeff has learned to take a deep breath and practice patience and compassion for Patrick and for himself during the morning chaos. Whenever he starts to feel tense, angry, or impatient, Jeff also asks himself, "Is my sense of panic and urgency necessary? Can I have empathy for Patrick and his ADHD right now? Can I have compassion for myself too?"

Related to an attitude of patience is an ability to show restraint. Together, patience and restraint are an antidote to impulsive actions. For example, one of my patients has a twenty-four-hour policy on buying things. When he or any of his family members see something exciting in a store, they have to wait twenty-four hours before actually purchasing it. Within that time, their initial emotions often die down and the purchase decision can be made in a more rational way.

Forgiveness

"I did not really learn to deal with my ADHD until I forgave myself." This startling statement came from Louise, an attractive, zippy woman in her forties. She was polished, gracious, and full of energy and charm—and I wondered why she would have to forgive herself. She explains: "As I look back on my life, there were times I got in my own way. I overreacted to things, misinterpreted situations, or did not look at my contribution to a problem. I tended to be high-strung, self-assured, and sometimes steamrolled others. I tended to be the joker and the star of the party, but missed out on the opportunities to truly be there for my friends." As she went through a list of regrets, she nonetheless emanated a sense of acceptance and forgiveness of herself. She said, "It took me a long time to come to terms with this, but forgiving myself has given me a certain peace I did not have before. It also helped me to change."

Willingness to Experience a Difficult Feeling

Kathy grew up on the East Coast but moved west during college. She ended up putting down roots in LA, while most of her immediate family remained back east. Kathy made regular trips to visit her family, which they appreciated but never reciprocated. Finally her brother Paul promised to visit one summer. Kathy was very much looking forward to it, wanting to show him the life she had created for herself. She took time off work that August in anticipation of his visit, and planned to take him to several places around town.

When August came, Paul called and told Kathy he wasn't going to visit after all. Instead he planned a trip with his family to Florida. Hearing the news Kathy told her brother, "No problem, I'll use my time off to take care of errands." She acted nonchalant, as if the change of plans didn't bother her. "Oh, well," she thought as she hung up the phone.

Later that evening, she felt a mounting feeling of disappointment and anger at her brother. She routinely pushed away such negative feelings, as she liked "being flexible" and "strong." This time, however, she allowed herself to feel the emotions with mindfulness. She watched them rise up, then fall, and then give way to a feeling of hurt as she thought about her family never visiting her. She noticed a strong urge to move away from the hurt, but she made a decision to be with the feeling. Tears welled up in her eyes, and she felt heaviness in her chest. She allowed herself to cry. She realized how tired she was of always making the effort to travel out east, and how much she wanted her family to come to visit her. She decided to call Paul the next day and talk to him about her feelings.

It's important to realize that when you first allow yourself to have a previously avoided feeling, it can be very intense, as if it's being expressed in a raw, childlike form. As an adult, it may feel embarrassing to have such a feeling, but it's important to see it as an intermediate stage of developing better emotional regulation. If you have avoided expressing anger, the first time you allow yourself to feel it, the emotion may be either very weak or very strong. If you try to communicate while you're angry, it may be clumsy or overreactive. It is important to be patient with yourself during this process. As you continue to allow yourself to experience the emotion with mindfulness, this difficulty generally improves—and what to say or do naturally becomes clear.

Willingness to Refrain from Acting on Emotion

Ian was going home after a long day at the office. He got in his car and headed for the parking lot exit, but it was blocked by another car. The woman in the car was a visitor and had gone to the wrong exit. A line of cars was forming behind her, and Ian realized he'd have to wait until the clog was cleared up. He started getting tense and felt a quick flash of rage. Normally, he'd start cursing and lay his fist on the car horn. This time, however, he said to himself, "Don't overreact," and decided to watch the rage with mindfulness. He took some breaths and labeled his feelings—"rage, rage, rage, rage"—until he felt the feeling diffuse a bit. He noted a shift in his reaction, which downgraded from rage to anger and impatience. He continued by labeling "anger, anger, anger" and then also noting "impatience, impatience, impatience." Being mindfully aware of the emotional reaction and labeling it with words helped him diffuse the reaction and diffuse the urge to act on his anger impulsively. He felt less tense, and he was proud of not "losing it."

The habit of indulging certain emotions can be fueled by certain thinking such as "I am right and you are wrong" or "I have a right to feel this way." While these statements may be true, they can at times fuel excessive negative emotions. Willingness to step back from the excessive feeling can help deal with the difficult situation. In intimate relationships, such willingness can foster communication and problem solving.

Positive Emotions

Cultivating positive emotions can counteract the burden of stress and negative emotions. The relatively new field of positive psychology has helped to emphasize how important positive emotions like gratitude or joy are in our lives.

The Science of Positive Psychology

Studies have shown that there are many benefits to positive emotions. For example:

- People tend to solve problems more creatively and with insight when they're in a positive mood. A positive mood appears to modulate attention and cognitive control areas of the brain and may enhance one's ability to come up with new solutions.[6]
- The practice of gratitude, in which one reviews daily events and gratefully appreciates helpful acts of others or the positive events of the day, has been shown to lift depression and promote joy and well-being.[7]
- In a classic study of Catholic nuns, the amount of joy, love, and hope expressed in a writing done in their twenties predicted their longevity. Those with a higher level of positive expression lived, on average, ten years longer than those with a lower level of such expression.[8]

Overall, the experience of positive emotions brings well-being and vitality. Here are a few suggestions to increase positive emotions in your life:

- Take time to make an inventory of your personal strengths. With ADHD there is much emphasis on negative symptoms and areas of struggle, so it's important to review the areas where you excel. What comes easily to you? What qualities you are proud of? As you list your strengths and positives, notice how you feel. Is it easy or hard to see yourself in a positive light? If you find yourself hesitating, ask your friends to help you name your strengths. Practice owning your strengths and actively bringing a sense of pride and gratitude for them.
- Seek out stories and books about successful adults with ADHD. These can bring hope and highlight creative solu-

tions for dealing with ADHD. They can help you reframe your own ADHD in a new, positive way.

- Practice gratitude at the end of each day. In difficult times, look for positive meaning to your difficulties—for example, being grateful for your resilience or lessons learned during a trying time.

- As you make your schedule or to-do list, include times for play or relaxation. If you have trouble taking time off because of a backlog of work, view the time off as a productive way to replenish your energy and be more effective when you return to work. Remember, playtime can also lead to a creative insight.

- Use laughter and humor daily—especially when dealing with your ADHD. Sometimes all you can do is laugh when you absentmindedly put your cookbook in the fridge or even when you forget to bring your ticket to a concert. Seek out ADHD humor online, in books, and at ADHD-related conferences and gatherings.

Suggested Reminders for Practice

- When thoughts and emotions are intense or difficult, use the RAIN steps:

  R = Recognize

  A = Accept

  I = Investigate

  N = Non-identify

  Post the RAIN steps in a place where you're likely to see them.

- Post loving-kindness wishes:

  May I be happy,
  May I be free of suffering,
  May I be safe,

May I peaceful and at ease,
May I find joy,
May I be healthy and strong,
May I accept myself as I am
May I...

....

Step 6 at a Glance

Formal Practice

- Do ten minutes (or more) of open-awareness meditation, such as the blue-sky meditation, each day. If you notice difficult thoughts or emotions, explore them with mindfulness, as in RAIN.
- Alternatively, do a ten-minute loving-kindness meditation each day.

Mindful Awareness in Daily Life

- Notice pleasant/unpleasant/neutral feelings in daily life. The table below can help you observe and label your feelings.[9] You can also use it to reflect on which emotions are generally common versus uncommon for you, or easy versus difficult for you.

Emotion Type	Specific Examples
Negative and forceful	Anger, Annoyance, Contempt, Disgust, Irritation
Negative and not in control	Anxiety, Embarrassment, Fear, Helplessness, Powerlessness, Worry
Negative thoughts	Doubt, Envy, Frustration, Guilt, Shame
Negative and passive	Boredom, Despair, Disappointment, Hurt, Sadness
Agitation	Stress, Shock, Tension

Emotion Type	Specific Examples
Positive and lively	Amusement, Delight, Elation, Excitement, Happiness, Joy, Pleasure
Caring	Affection, Empathy, Friendliness, Love
Positive thoughts	Courage, Hope, Pride, Satisfaction, Trust
Quiet positive	Calm, Content, Relaxed, Relieved, Serene
Reactive	Interest, Politeness, Surprise

- Use STOP or RAIN practices to enhance awareness of emotions in daily life.
- Pause for loving-kindness whenever you're experiencing difficult emotions.
- Practice attitudes of self-compassion, forgiveness, patience, and willingness in daily life.
- Increase positive emotions including humor, playfulness, and gratitude. Try keeping a gratitude journal where you record one to three things you are grateful for each day.

STEP 7   Communicate Skillfully

Mindful Listening and Speaking

Joan has always been high-energy and high-strung. Her sister Molly describes her as "difficult to be around." Molly says, "It's hard to just have a simple conversation with Joan. She interrupts a lot and quickly gets intense. It's as if she constantly has to prove her point. She also asks a lot of questions, which I find very annoying and also kind of aggressive, but she says, 'I'm just curious.' At one point, even her boss told her she asked too many questions." During our appointment I asked Joan about this, and she simply replied, "My boss is rude." She didn't see a problem.

Difficulties in communication and social skills are common in children with ADHD and often continue into their adulthood. Pitfalls like interrupting or not listening are so common in ADHD that they are used to diagnose it. There are also often difficulties with clear, direct, and *appropriately* assertive communication, which leads to impulsive or emotionally charged conversations, arguments, and others' discomfort. Although not always recognized by adults with ADHD as something they need to work on, these problems can lead to frustration, feeling misunderstood, or a sense of isolation. In marriages where one or both partners have ADHD, we often find high conflict, stress, and a history of divorce.

In this step, we focus on mindful communication. Here you'll observe your communication style and practice mindful listening and speaking.

ADHD and Common Communication Pitfalls

You may not be aware of how your communication is received by others. Below is a list of common communication problems in ADHD. Try to review them with a nonjudgmental attitude, and check the ones that apply to you. Then have your spouse, a family member, or a friend give you their view.

INATTENTION CAN LEAD TO:
- ❏ Tuning out part of a conversation.
- ❏ Being told you don't listen.
- ❏ Forgetting what was said.
- ❏ Feeling lost in a conversation.

IMPULSIVITY CAN LEAD TO:
- ❏ Interrupting
- ❏ Impatience in a conversation
- ❏ Talking too much
- ❏ Talking too loudly
- ❏ Blurting things out
- ❏ Saying something you later regret

EXECUTIVE FUNCTION DIFFICULTIES CAN LEAD TO:
- ❏ A tendency to go off topic
- ❏ Giving too much detail in a conversation (for example, storytelling when a quick answer is called for)
- ❏ Repetition
- ❏ Saying the same thing, but in a different way
- ❏ Jumping from one topic to another
- ❏ Communicating in a disorganized way, leading to confused or lost listeners

EMOTIONAL REGULATION PROBLEMS AND
LOW SELF-ESTEEM CAN LEAD TO:

☐ Being flooded with emotion but being unable to verbally express it.
☐ Excessive anger.
☐ Being overly sensitive to criticism.
☐ Trying to be overly pleasing—having trouble saying "no" or disagreeing.
☐ Being oppositional—having trouble saying "yes" or agreeing.

Observing Your Own Communication

Think about your day-to-day conversations. Many times, if you follow the content and flow of the words, you can imagine a conversation as moving in a kind of line. But those lines can be very different for those who have ADHD and those who don't.

The following example demonstrates this disparity. The lines represent the flow of the two responses.

Conversation with Jim, an Adult with ADHD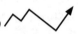

Doctor: How's the new job going?

Jim: I got there the first day and the woman giving orientation was so slow and boring I thought I'd jump out of my skin. I had to excuse myself and get some coffee. You know, I'm drinking more coffee lately and not sure if that means my stimulant isn't working. I start my morning with an espresso and usually have at least two other cups during the day. But I'd like to cut it. In general I'm trying to exercise more and eat better. My wife wants me to lose weight.

Doctor: So going back to the job, how are you doing *there?*

Conversation with Robert, an Adult without ADHD ⟶

Doctor: How's the new job going?

Robert: Good. I'm still getting used to the new schedule, but overall I like it.

Jim wasn't aware of how his response veered off subject. If he'd been able to catch himself veering off sooner or make a conscious decision to remember the original question, he could have self-corrected. This ability can be developed through mindfulness practice.

EXPLORATION 7.1
STOP as You Talk

You can use the versatile STOP reminder to develop more awareness of your conversations and aid in directing the flow of your words. As you talk, imagine part of you standing aside, monitoring your exchanges with curiosity.

S = *Stop* and unhook from being on automatic pilot

T = *Take a mindful breath*

O = *Observe* how the conversation is going and where you are in the process. You can ask yourself the following questions:
- Where is my attention?
- Am I focused on the speaker and the original question or topic?
- Is my body relaxed or tense?
- What inner thoughts and feelings am I aware of as I speak?
- What attitude do I have right now? (Judgmental, nonjudgmental?)
- Is there an urge to interrupt when the other person is speaking?

P = *Proceed,* either by continuing as you were or by correcting aspects of your experience:
- If you're distracted, refocus on the speaker.
- If you're going off topic or "branching out," return to the original topic.
- If you're tense, relax your body.

- If you're feeling reactive or overly emotional, label the feeling and try to take deep breaths to calm your body and mind. Sometimes it may help to acknowledge to the other person how you're feeling, such as, "I'm getting flustered as we talk about this."
- If you feel judgmental, try to adopt a nonjudgmental attitude and tone.
- If you're interrupting or have the urge to interrupt, notice it and try to withhold the response.

Notes about Observing Your Communication

Use the STOP practice in different social situations—for example, talking to friends, talking to your boss. Be curious about the difference in how you and your communication are in each context.

If you notice that you space out while conversing, try asking the person to repeat what he or she just said. Be honest; don't pretend you know what they said. If the relationship is close, you can let them know your mind wandered off because of your ADHD. Usually the person won't have a problem repeating the information and will appreciate that you really want to be attentive.

Use strategies that help you stay alert and focused. For example, shift or straighten your body and refocus on the other person's eyes. Or try using nonobtrusive strategies that give you additional stimulation—for example, wiggle your toes, play with a paperclip, or doodle discreetly. The latter strategies are also helpful if restlessness makes it hard to listen.

From time to time, renew the intention to be more present to the other person. Remind yourself that true listening is a gift we can offer each other.

Check for Sensitivity to Criticism

Emotional sensitivity is often reported by adults with ADHD and may include being oversensitive to criticism. The latter

MINDFULNESS FOR ADHD

can especially hinder communication by making an adult with ADHD overreact or quickly become defensive in conversations. And once a negative feeling is evoked, it can be difficult to control or "dial down" the emotion. So as you observe your communication, notice the instances of receiving feedback or criticism with renewed curiosity and study your typical reaction. Check for the following:

- Do you dismiss the criticism immediately?
- Is there intense hurt or anger?
- Is there shame or "feeling down on yourself"?
- Do you tell yourself, "I'm too sensitive"?
- Do you quickly blame the other person or think things like, "You're such a jerk"?

Practice noticing your reaction with some distance and use strategies to manage the sensitivity. For example:

- If intense hurt or shame is evoked, practice self-compassion and loving-kindness. It can also help to remind yourself, "Hearing criticism is hard for me."
- If judgmental or negative thoughts about yourself arise because of the criticism, observe them with mindfulness. For example, if you notice thoughts like "I'm a failure," remind yourself this is only a thought. Think of the blue-sky-and-clouds metaphor to step back from such judgmental thinking. Also practice accepting yourself even if the criticism is true. Ask: "Can I accept myself even in this very moment?" Remember the criticism doesn't have to diminish your sense of worth; you can look at it objectively and learn from it.
- If you tend to quickly dismiss criticism, be open to considering it. Is there some truth to the criticism? Take what's useful. Ask others their opinion to help you assess if the criticism is accurate.
- Finally, notice if your reaction to criticism differs depending on who is delivering it. Such selective sensitivity may

be a signal that something else (such as previous disappointments or anger) is creating obstacles in the relationship.

Communication in Relationships

Communication plays an important role in relationships, and adults with ADHD often have difficulties in this domain. ADHD-related communication problems can create tension and hurt feelings between partners, coworkers, and friends, especially if the behaviors are seen as intentional or attributed to not caring. In addition, ADHD adults with problems managing emotions or a tendency to be oppositional may be quick-tempered, frequently blaming others, or becoming defensive in conversations. Disorganization, lateness, and a lack of follow-through can also become a point of contention and frustration for others, especially if repeated requests for change don't lead to improvement. Finally, since ADHD can also get in the way of recognizing and expressing one's own feelings and needs, achieving true intimacy in romantic relationships may be difficult. In this section we look at mindful practices and perspectives that foster better communication with others.

EXPLORATION 7.2
Mindful Listening and Speaking

This exercise involves speaking slowly and taking turns. It's usually done in pairs, and is a good practice for romantic partners who want to develop better communication skills.

- Start by sitting across from your partner. Practice a relaxed and receptive posture (for example, lean slightly forward, and avoid crossing your arms) and maintain frequent, natural eye contact.
- Pick a topic that is meaningful, or problematic, or both,

MINDFULNESS FOR ADHD

for both of you (such as, Where are we going for holidays this year?).

- Have one of you be solely the speaker and the other solely the listener for thirty seconds. Then switch. Take turns speaking and listening in this manner for five or ten minutes or until you exhaust the topic. Use a timer if you have trouble keeping to the thirty-second intervals. This is good practice in time awareness, too.

WHEN MINDFULLY LISTENING — LISTEN FULLY
- Listen with full attention.
- Withhold an impulse to interrupt or give feedback.
- Practice being open, empathetic, and nonjudgmental.
- Breathe, relax your body, and continue.

WHEN MINDFULLY SPEAKING — SPEAK WITH AWARENESS
- Speak more slowly than usual, choosing your words thoughtfully.
- Practice speaking from the heart: being honest, direct, and vulnerable.
- Breathe, relax your body, and continue.

Nonviolent Communication

Another tool for mindful communication is called *nonviolent* (or *compassionate*) *communication* developed by the psychologist Marshall Rosenberg and explained in depth in his 2003 book, *Nonviolent Communication: A Language of Life*. The steps involved in nonviolent communication help express feelings and needs in a relationship, because when feelings and needs are not addressed, they often fuel a problem. The inherently compassionate approach of nonviolent communication is not always intuitive, especially when negative emotions and conflict are high. So next time there is a problem you want to address with another person, practice the following four steps:

1. *Observe* the facts nonjudgmentally (for example, "When…").
2. Express your *feelings* evoked by the observations (for example, "I feel…").
3. Express your *needs* related to these feelings (for example, "It's because I need…").
4. Make a specific *request* of another person (for example, "I would like…").

For example, Anne explains to her husband, "When you ask me if I paid the monthly bills [observation], I often have a sinking feeling just thinking about it [feelings]. Because of my ADHD, keeping up with mail and paperwork is really difficult for me and I need help with it [need]. Could you help me keep track of the bills? [request]"

Compare this to, "Why do you keep nagging me about the bills?! Why don't you just do it!"

The steps of nonviolent communication can also help convey empathy for the other person. In this case, you also observe the facts nonjudgmentally, but instead of your own feelings, reflect on the other person's experience and offer your impressions of which of their needs may not be addressed. In this process you may be making some guesses about the other person's feelings and needs. Propose these in a nonjudgmental and inquisitive way to create an opening for more empathic dialogue. The request step is usually omitted here.

For example, Andrew expresses empathy with his wife: "When I forgot our anniversary [observation], you probably felt frustrated and ignored [feeling]. And you want a relationship where you feel important and cared about [need]."

Compare that to, "Sorry I forgot the anniversary, but you don't have to be so sensitive about it."

Developing Empathy in Relationships Affected by ADHD

Practicing mindful communication can help resolve misunderstandings, frustration, and conflicts. However, educating family members and friends about ADHD symptoms and their effects on relationships is crucial for creating mutual understanding and empathy. Consider this example for marital therapy:

Judy and Mark have been married for five years. Judy complains that Mark often forgets things they discuss and acts as if she never talked to him about them. She feels ignored and frustrated by his seeming lack of care. She thinks he does this on purpose because "other things are more important to him." Mark accuses Judy of being critical and nagging. He says that she reads too much into his forgetting, which is usually accidental on his part. Overall he thinks, "It's not a big deal."

As the therapy progresses, it's clear that Mark has ADHD symptoms. His forgetfulness is significant but not an intentional act of ignoring Judy. Education about ADHD helps Judy and Mark have a new understanding and empathy for their difficulties. The new perspective does not solve their issues, but it creates a critical shift toward acceptance and mutual problem-solving. Judy learns to take the forgetfulness less personally and to be less critical and more compassionate. Mark learns to take responsibility for his forgetfulness and be more understanding of the impact it can have on Judy. They both practice mindful speaking and listening in therapy sessions and at home. Judy makes eye contact with Mark when she tells him something important and often gives him gentle reminders. He practices focusing on her fully whenever she speaks and starts to write things down in a personal organizer to help him remember things. Overall, he is less defensive and more proactive in solving the issue, and Judy is more understanding and helpful in mitigating the ADHD pitfalls. They both are more supportive of each other and now can even joke about Mark's ADHD moments.

Mindfulness can enhance the goodwill created by ADHD education. For example, Judy uses mindfulness to modulate the frustration that crops up whenever Mark still forgets something. Mark uses mindful breathing to step back from annoyance that arises when Judy reminds him about something. Both also started a practice of loving-kindness, in which they send the wishes of well-being to themselves and to each other. They challenge themselves to do this practice even if—and especially when—one of them is hurt or angry. This practice of acting in a way that is contrary to your immediate feelings is not easy and requires a conscious decision; however, it often creates a positive emotional shift. It can help you connect with feelings of love and generosity for your partner, even in the midst of conflict, and open up the potential for mindful communication.

For more on the topic of relationships and ADHD, check out the books *Is It You, Me, or Adult ADD?* (2008), by Gina Pera, and *The ADHD Effect on Marriage* (2010), by Melissa Orlov.

ADHD and Parenting

Frustrations and misunderstandings can also arise in the parent-child relationship. ADHD shows strong familial predisposition, and adults with ADHD often have children with ADHD, too. Such a combination can be especially challenging, as both the parent and the child may be struggling with disorganization, negative emotions, and stress.

Research has shown that the brain maturity of children with ADHD tends to be delayed by about three years; thus on average an eleven-year-old with ADHD has a maturity level that is more similar to the maturity level of a non-ADHD eight-year-old.[1] In daily life, this means that ADHD children often have trouble modulating their behavior even though they may be expected to do so in school and at home. They also may have less frustration tolerance and show delays in learning. That can lead to tension and misunderstandings in their relationship with parents.

If you are a parent of a child with ADHD, remember that your child is struggling in ways that may not be readily apparent. As a parent, you are a teacher, and how you approach your children has tremendous impact on them. With mindfulness, you can communicate nonjudgmental and compassionate observations of your child's ADHD and model such perspective to him or her. You can help your child develop self-acceptance and encourage positive ways for them to cope with their difficulties. You can also teach your child mindfulness directly. (See the concluding chapter for mindfulness resources for kids.)

Finally, when the stress of parenting gets to you, use mindfulness to help you deal with negative feelings. Find a moment of respite, and practice self-compassion. After all, parenting is hard and no parent is perfect. With mindfulness you can transform difficult moments to moments of learning and insight.

For more on using mindfulness to deal with parenting stress, see *The Family ADHD Solution* (2011), by the pediatrician Mark Bertin.

Mindful Presence: Choiceless Awareness

The ability to be fully present to yourself and another person requires a flexible and receptive attention. It calls for the ability to be aware of whatever arises from moment to moment in an interaction. This ability—awareness of the changing flow of experience within us and outside of us—is strengthened by the practice on track 9 of the CD, "Mindful Presence," also called *choiceless awareness*.

In this practice we don't choose a specific object to focus on; instead we practice receiving the flow of present-moment experience, whatever shape it takes.

EXPLORATION 7.3
Mindful Presence (CD track 9; ten minutes)

GET SETTLED AND RELAXED
- Sit comfortably in an upright position.
- Briefly scan your body and relax any areas of tension.

ANCHOR ATTENTION ON THE BREATH
- Gently rest your attention on the breath. Feel the gentle movement of your breath at the nostrils, abdomen, or chest.

- Remember, the breath is always there, always in the present. You can always return to it if you get lost in thinking or feeling.

SET YOUR INTENTION
- Set the intention to be aware and receptive to whatever arises in each moment.
- Notice where your attention goes—if something strongly pulls it, investigate that, then return to the breath.
  - If a *sound* becomes obvious, open up your attention to allow awareness of that sound alongside the breathing. If the sound pulls your attention away from the breath, place your full attention on the sound and allow the breathing sensations to fall into the background. Listen to the sound until it no longer holds your attention. Then return to the breath.
  - If a *body sensation* arises, open up your attention to it and hold both the sensation and your breathing together in awareness. If the sensation pulls your attention away from the breath, turn your attention to it and allow the breath to fade into the background. Explore the sensation: Is it itching, burning? Does it stay the same or is it changing? When it no longer holds your attention, again return to breathing, the anchor of awareness.
  - If an *emotion* becomes obvious, as with other experiences, open your attention to and notice it alongside of your breathing. If the emotion pulls your attention, then focus on it and allow the breath to fade into the background. You can use the RAIN practice to observe the emotion: recognize and accept, then investigate and don't identify with it. Label the emotion and check into your body. Maybe there is fluttering or uneasiness in the belly. When the emotion is no longer present, bring your attention back to

the breath and whatever else may be obvious in the present moment.

- ○ If a *thought or image* comes to your awareness, acknowledge its presence as you continue breathing. Many times, thoughts remain in the background and you can be aware of them coming and going, like clouds in the sky. If you get lost in thinking, once you notice the lapse of awareness, label it as "thinking" and gently return to the breath. If a thought is obsessive and keeps coming back, bring your attention to it and allow the breath to fade into the background. Label the type of thought, such as "worrying," "planning," or "judgmental thought." Check in to the body and see if there are any emotions or body sensations present. When ready, return your attention back to the breath.
- ○ You may also notice other things. Maybe a general state of energy, alertness level, or an attitude or mood. You can investigate each experience until you are ready to notice the next one.

END WITH APPRECIATION AND LOVING-KINDNESS

- Give yourself appreciation for sitting through this practice of awareness. Extend *loving-kindness* to yourself and wish yourself well—for example, "May I be happy, may I be safe, may I be healthy and live with ease. May I be present to myself and others."
- Extend these wishes to all people—such as, "May we all be happy, safe, healthy, and at ease. May we all experience true listening and empathy in each other."

Suggested Reminders for Practice

A reminder sign to STOP is helpful when working with this step of the program:

- S = Stop
- T = Take a breath
- O = Observe speaking and listening
- P = Proceed

....

Step 7 at a Glance

Formal Practices

- Do a fifteen-minute sitting practice of mindful presence (CD track 9) each day.
- Alternatively, you can do a fifteen-minute walking meditation, noting all of your experiences.

Mindful Awareness in Daily Life

- Practice STOP in interactions with others at work and home.
- Practice mindful listening and speaking with your partner or your child, using the following forms of expression:
  1. Slow speaking, taking turns
  2. Nonviolent/compassionate communication: "When..." *(observe the facts)*, "I feel..." *(feeling)*. "It's because..." *(need)*. "I'd like..." *(request)*.
- Try an improvisation workshop. In such workshops you have to be constantly attentive to what is happening from moment to moment in order to quickly respond. This can make you more aware of your thoughts, feelings, and responses.

Slow Down to Be More Effective

Mindful Decisions and Actions

Joan struggles with disorganization. She has trouble keeping track of her two elementary school–age kids' activities, and her house is messy and cluttered. She says she has "piles of stuff" in the closet, and her desk has bills, junk mail, magazines, and kids' school notes all mixed in together. She often can't find things. Yet she procrastinates on her now six-month project of organizing the desk. "I really want to be more organized," she says. "I even bought a new file cabinet . . . but I haven't been able to actually use it."

Kirk has a different problem. He likes to tinker and tends to have many simultaneous household projects. He recently started to redo the fence in the garden. He got it mostly done, but without finishing it he moved on to fixing his garage door. His wife complains that he has trouble wrapping things up. Kirk is aware that this is a problem, and he promises to finish the fence, but he keeps working on the garage — and now has even started to tinker with his car.

It's often said that adults with ADHD know what to do — they just can't get it done. Joan knows she needs to organize her desk, but she still procrastinates. Kirk knows he has too many projects, but he still starts a new one before completing the ones in progress. There's a disconnection between understanding and action.

In this chapter, we'll bridge this gap by putting together the mindfulness tools you learned in steps 1–7. You'll practice deepening your awareness of what's happening to you at each stage of a task, from start to finish. Such awareness leads to mindful self-coaching: an inner voice that can help guide your actions. Used together with organizational tools like a calendar and to-do list, this self-coaching voice will help you make mindful decisions and get things done.

Mindfulness of Actions

In the previous steps, we talked about awareness of the body, thoughts, and emotions. These inner experiences come together to direct our behavior. They're powerful motivators—and powerful barriers—to achieving our goals. Mindfulness helps us discern what's happening inside us with more clarity and allows us to shape our decisions and actions so they can work *for* us—not against us. With mindfulness, we often also find inner resources we didn't think we had.

Q: I'm already aware that I'm procrastinating. Will mindful awareness help me get things done?

While you may be aware that you're procrastinating, you may not be aware of the deeper thoughts or feelings that drive that procrastination. Or you may be unsure about how to shift out of procrastination and motivate yourself into *doing*. Mindful awareness can help you develop a greater ability to *turn toward the avoidance of doing*, as it's happening. You learn to label this avoidance in the moment and observe nonjudgmentally your inner barriers (negative thoughts and feelings toward the task). You can also, in that moment, choose to increase the inner motivations for doing the task. Such awareness is often a key in overcoming procrastination as it's happening, and it can help you utilize additional tools—like a planner, cognitive behavioral therapy, or coaching—to keep you on track.

The three basic principles in using mindfulness with actions are:

- Pausing
- Practicing calm focus
- Mindful self-coaching

Let's focus on each one of these more closely.

Pausing

During the course of your day, it is helpful to periodically pause and "take stock" of your actions and how you're addressing the tasks that need to be done. The familiar STOP practice can be helpful here.

EXPLORATION 8.1
Using the STOP Practice with Tasks

As you tackle your work, use STOP to look more deeply into your attention, body, thoughts, feelings, and behavior.

*S*top for a moment

*T*ake a breath

*O*bserve in the present moment:
- Is there good interest and motivation?
- Is there boredom and lack of motivation?
- Is there avoidance or procrastination?
- Is there high or low energy?
- Is there a feeling or thought (or both) of being over-whelmed, or is there a sense of empowerment?
- Is there doubt (for example, "Should I be doing this?")
- Is there a feeling of wanting to do something else?

- Am I *already doing something else?* (Doing something that's productive but not the task you planned on is a sneaky way to procrastinate.)
- Whatever you find, bring your full attention to it. Check in to your body a little more and notice any other thoughts and feelings that may be there (for example, "My chest is heavy" or "My mind is sharp"). If you notice an obstacle to doing your task, imagine you're looking directly at the obstacle and name it in your mind—for example, "Oh, there's avoidance."
- You may also find that obstacles are easier to conquer if you say them aloud or write them on a piece of paper. You can also call a friend and share with them: "I've been procrastinating about this." Often full acknowledgment in a mindful, nonjudgmental way can diminish the power of the obstacle and re-motivate you for the task.

Proceed with new awareness.

Calm Focus

Calm focus is necessary to do any work effectively. If you're anxious, frazzled, or frustrated, these feelings will make it extra challenging to focus or get organized. You're more likely to make mistakes, omit important details, or not see an obvious solution.

If at any point in your day you notice being overwhelmed, uneasy, agitated, or restlessness, practice calming your body and mind. Try the following:

• Take several deep, mindful breaths; do a short sitting meditation focusing on the breath; or do a body scan to induce calm and shift your perspective.

- Use imagery and meditation together to feel calmer and more focused. You can use the "Mind Like an Ocean" meditation from step 5 or try the Mountain Meditation below, which cultivates calm focus and inner stability.

EXPLORATION 8.2
The Mountain Meditation

- Sit in an upright posture but without strain: a posture of dignity.
- Allow yourself to just sit and notice your breathing.
- Imagine a mountain, and reflect on how strong and solid it is.
- Reflect on how the mountain is connected to the earth and has been standing there for thousands of years through rain, snow, wind, or sun.
- Now imagine yourself as that mountain. Connect with a feeling of being solid and strong in your body's core.
- Like a mountain, you can be grounded no matter what swirls around you. You can watch an overwhelming feeling pass by you like rainy clouds passing the mountain.
- As you sit, bring awareness to your breathing and silently repeat the following words:

  "Breathing in, I see myself like a mountain."

  "Breathing out, I feel solid and strong."

- After a while, as you breathe simply say in your mind:

  "In...mountain"

  "Out...solid and strong"

- Repeat the phrases in your mind until you feel solid, strong, and less overwhelmed.

If you like this practice, find a picture of a mountain (or draw one) and keep it posted in your workspace. It can be a visual reminder of your solid, inner strength as you tackle each stage of your tasks.

Mindful Self-Coaching

Through mindfulness we can fine-tune our inner self-talk to help us become more efficient and effective. This voice, which I call the *mindful self-coaching* voice, is typically unreliable in ADHD adults, who often depend on external forces to get a project done. For example, adults with ADHD often procrastinate until there's a deadline or another person to motivate them.

Mindfulness, however, can help you develop this self-coaching voice to guide your actions from within, including doing tasks that are difficult for you. I believe a simultaneous fine-tuning of this internal voice along with wise use of external tools, such as a calendar, a to-do list, reminders, or medication, is most helpful in ADHD.

Mindful self-coaching involves developing a supportive, compassionate, and encouraging inner voice that is also informed by frequent checking in to the present moment. Some examples: "This is hard for me but I know I can do it," "I'll keep trying," "I need to slow down," or "I need to pick up the pace." As you practice mindfulness and experience deeper awareness of yourself and others, you build a reservoir of insight and discernment that can further guide your actions.

Strategies for Getting Things Done

We now take a look how you can use pausing, calm focus, and mindful self-coaching to be more effective in day-to-day tasks. Getting things done, together with managing time, is a challenge for many ADHD adults. The mindful approach to completing tasks invites you to develop a habit of monitoring how you are doing throughout the task sequence of choosing, starting, doing, and finishing. By being more present at each stage—even if what you're doing is avoidance of the task—you develop a greater ability for choice, self-regulation, and mindful action; in short, getting the job done.

Choose, Start, Do, and Finish Tasks with Mindfulness

Check in to the present moment and deepen awareness of your inner state and actions at each stage of a task.

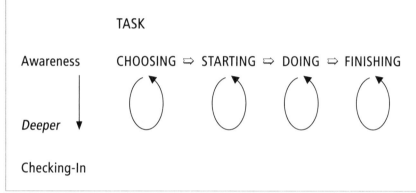

Choosing a Task

Many of our lives are filled with simultaneous things we could be doing on any given day or at any given time. Knowing where to put your energies can be challenging. It can be even more daunting with ADHD, since having an ADHD brain can mean having many ideas but a poor ability to organize them. Many adults with ADHD report being overwhelmed by their choices and not knowing where to start. Others may be driven by distractions while overlooking important tasks. Many are constantly busy—but ineffective. A majority find it hard to keep their focus on important goals, especially goals that reach far into the future. Instead, immediate things often take over and steal their attention and energy. To counteract this, it is important for adults with ADHD to periodically stop and take stock of the big picture.

A mindfulness-based approach called Acceptance Commitment Therapy (ACT), created by psychologist and researcher Steven Hayes,[1] offers a useful way to help us reflect on our values so that we can choose actions mindfully. Values are the principles that guide our life and action. They are different from goals or outcomes in that they are not something we achieve and move on from. Rather, they are guiding standards—for example, having the value of "being a good athlete," in contrast to having the goal of "winning the next game"; the value of "being physically fit," versus the goal of "losing ten pounds."

When clarifying your values in several areas of your life—work, relationships, social life, hobbies—you can also check how much time you're actually devoting to each. This is often an eye-opening experience. For example, even if being a good parent is an important value, you may be spending only a small fraction of your weekly time with your children. Thus, there's a misalignment between your values and your actual behavior. For each area, you also identify actions that you can do now to rebalance your life. Such reflection can help you decide where and when you want to put your energies and identify what steps you should take next. Reflecting on your values also helps you simplify your life and notice what really matters.

Below is a worksheet to help you identify your values in ten important life domains. I encourage you to fill it out even if it seems tedious. Making your values explicit and external gives you a solid anchor to come back to if you need to refocus or reprioritize in the future.

As you complete the table, keep in mind that even if you find an area where you haven't been doing well, this is your chance to start mending that. Also realize that you can only do one thing at a time well. When you have a block of time, choose only one value and do something toward fulfilling it, however small it is. Having a balanced life doesn't mean being perfect in each life domain. It simply means being able to keep up with important things in your life on a regular basis.

EXPLORATION 8.3
Values Worksheet

- In each life domain (first column), write one important value. There may be more than one value you can think of for each domain, but just start with one that seems especially significant.
- In columns A and B, reflect on your life in a nonjudgmental way.

Column A: Rate how important the value is to you on a scale of 1 to 10 (with 1 being "not important at all" and 10 being "extremely important").

Column B: On a scale of 1 to 10, how important does this value seem to be as demonstrated by your actual behavior?

Column C: Come up with one short-term and one long-term goal that can help you bring your actions in line with your values.

Life Domain/My Value	A	B	C
	Importance of this value 1-10	Rating according to my actual behavior 1-10	ST = short term goals LT = long term goals
example: Health/Well-Being *Manage my ADHD well*	9	3	ST: *Get an evaluation*
			LT: *Read books or websites describing available tools for adult ADHD*

You can download a printable version of this table from www.shambhala.com/MindfulnessPrescription.

Life Domain/My Value	A	B	C
	Importance of this value 1-10	Rating according to my actual behavior 1-10	ST = short term goals LT = long term goals
Health/Well-Being			ST:
			LT:
Intimate Relationship			ST:
			LT:
Parenting			ST:
			LT:
Family Relationships			ST:
			LT:
Friendship/Social			ST:
			LT:
Career/Work			ST:
			LT:

Life Domain/My Value	A	B	C
	Importance of this value 1-10	Rating according to my actual behavior 1-10	ST = short term goals LT = long term goals
Education/Personal Growth			ST:
			LT:
Recreation/Leisure			ST:
			LT:
Spirituality			ST:
			LT:
Citizenship			ST:
			LT:

Starting a Task

When you plan on tackling an important daily task or addressing one of your value-related goals, try some of the following strategies:

- Find and jump-start your motivation.
- Develop your engine.
- Use music.

- Watch your willingness or lack of it.
- Notice basic feelings: pleasant, unpleasant, and neutral.
- Start the task "sideways" versus "head on."

FIND AND JUMP-START YOUR MOTIVATION

Some adults develop inner motivation strategies like self-criticism that do motivate them, but at a cost. Here's an example: Chris is a fairly successful cabinetmaker in his forties. He has ADHD but also struggles with anxiety and depression. He is very critical of himself and often downplays his accomplishments, seeming to always find some way in which he is lacking. When I point out his achievements, he says, "I'm afraid that if I start giving myself credit for what I've done, I'm going to lose my engine. If I stop criticizing myself, I may get lazy and slack off." While this never-be-satisfied-with-myself inner voice has been driving his performance, the same voice robs Chris of enjoyment in life. He can't relax during his time off and constantly worries he should be doing more.

It's important for adults with ADHD to self-motivate without using the critical voice. Instead, inner motivation can often become stronger by finding a larger meaning to the task at hand. A well-known story illustrates this point:

Three men are working side by side. A passerby asks the first worker, "What are you doing?" The first worker says, "I'm moving bricks."

The passerby asks the second worker the same question. The second worker answers, "I'm building a wall."

Then the passerby addresses the third worker, asking, "And what are you doing?" The third worker replies, "I'm building a cathedral."

Through self-coaching we can think like the third worker, finding a positive way to mentally frame each task. While negative consequences can be powerful motivators—for example, getting repeated speeding tickets can make you drive more slowly—see if you can find your own *positive* reasons for doing the right thing ("I want to be a safe driver"). Be curious about what motivates you more: a positive framing of the task or thinking of the negative consequences?

Jump-start your motivation by imagining the outcome. For example, envision having a clear desk and how it would feel to have removed the burden of piles of messy papers. Really savor this image and try to notice the body sensations, thoughts, and feelings it evokes. Finally, say your motivation aloud or write it down in a place you can see it.

Finally, remember that by following through with your chosen task, no matter how small, you're training yourself to develop the inner muscle to self-direct.

REV YOUR ENGINE

If you're having trouble getting started, your energy may be too low and you may need to raise it. Physical exercise is great for that, but you can also try a brief meditation with imagery that gets you to be mobilized and motivated. Let's try it.

EXPLORATION 8.4
"Breathing In, I Am Like..."

- Think of an image from nature, your life, books, or a movie that helps you connect with readiness to *focus and take action*—for example, a crouching tiger or a diver getting ready to jump.
- Now imagine yourself being that focused and ready to act. Create your own meditation by completing this phrase:

  Breathing in, I am like a _____ (insert your image).

  Breathing out, I am _____ (insert the quality you want).

For example:

   Breathing in, I see myself as a tiger.

   Breathing out, I am focused and ready to act.

Or in short:

In ~ tiger

Out ~ ready to act

- Breathe and repeat the phrase several times. See if you can connect with the sense of raising energy and motivation in your body. See if you can sense your willingness and readiness to tackle the task.

The tiger image helps me when I'm procrastinating. Sometimes I even add the words "Jump tiger!" to help me tackle my task. I see this imagery as effective, but also playful and funny. The playful part reminds me not to take the task and the procrastination too seriously and just get started.

USE MUSIC

Music can have a powerful effect on the mind and body. As you approach an unpleasant task, put on some music that you know usually perks you up. Perhaps you'll notice a rising urge to tap your foot or move your body to the rhythm. You might have an increased sense of energy and "outgoingness." Maybe you'll notice both tiredness and an inner energy together. Focus on feelings of playfulness and motivation brought about by the music. Embrace these feelings, and choose to amplify them in your body. Is there more ease in tackling the unpleasant task now?

Alternatively, you can put on calming music. Such music, often used in spas, can help shift your body and mind into a relaxed mode. Bring mindful awareness to this process and notice any thoughts, feelings, or body sensations present. Ask yourself: "Is it easier to tackle a task when I am relaxed or energized?"

Always be clear and honest about whether you want or don't want to do something. Here's an example: Kelly, a hairdresser, was reflecting on her business. "My salon is slowing down," she said, "yet I don't feel like putting any effort into marketing it. I know this isn't a good decision in the long run, but right now I just don't feel like I want to do anything about it." Kelly's statement is refreshingly honest. In our culture of industriousness, to admit reluctance to do anything can be hard.

Acknowledging this lack of will without guilt or stress is a step of acceptance. It's a statement of "this is what it is." After such honest acknowledgment, though, often there's an opening for a follow-up question, such as: "Do I want to change this?" Sometimes the answer may still be no. It's an honest declaration and allows you the freedom to consciously decide to walk away from a task. This process also leads to the freedom to later decide to put the effort in.

NOTICE THE BASIC FEELINGS—PLEASANT, UNPLEASANT, AND NEUTRAL

As you have already explored, virtually all our life experiences can be described by three basic feelings: "I like it" (pleasant); "I don't like it" (unpleasant); and "I don't feel much about it" (neutral). These basic feelings can drive many of our choices, often without our full awareness. For adults with ADHD, it's often difficult to stay with an unpleasant or neutral (boring) task. Yet life often requires it. There is a concept, attributed to the psychologist John Lehnhoff,[2] the "hate-it-but-do-it center" of the mind, which describes the self-coaching part of us, willing to endure discomfort because something is meaningful or important. I think this phrase and the concept behind it are very useful when dealing with ADHD symptoms. The hate-it-but-do-it center is a cornerstone of self-discipline. With mindfulness, the feelings of discomfort and intense dislike of the situation, as well as willingness, can be watched with curiosity.

Sometimes it may feel overwhelming to start a task head-on. Instead, try starting it "sideways"—beginning with a small aspect of the task or telling yourself "I don't have to do the entire thing, I can just peek at it." Sometimes "peeking" into a project lowers the anxiety of starting it. Once you are engaged in the task, you may find that it isn't so hard, and your hyperfocus can keep you going. Be aware of your body as you think of starting the task "head on" versus "sideways"; see if you notice a difference.

Doing a Task

Once you have started a task, here some ways to keep you staying with it:

- Make a list, prioritize, and break tasks down.
- Focus on one thing at a time and keep coming back after a distraction.
- If you multitask, do it with mindfulness.
- Keep encouraging yourself.
- Watch and vary your pace.
- Take breaks, but watch for the tendency to extend them.
- Look for help from "external engines," structures, or people.

MAKE A LIST, PRIORITIZE, AND BREAK TASKS DOWN

The basic strategies of organization—listing, ranking, and breaking tasks down on paper—are a must for those with ADHD. These strategies support the executive function skills, which as we know with ADHD are weak. They are also especially helpful when, at any point, you notice a sense of being overwhelmed, having a "brain freeze," or being lost within a task. If so, write a to-do list, rank the items on the list in order of importance, and break the big jobs down into smaller chunks. Doing this is often like giving your brain "a sigh of relief." After all, you're freeing up your brain from having to remember everything throughout your task.

You can also draw the information (make a chart or table), use flash cards with steps and lay them out, or talk it through out aloud. Notice with mindfulness what organizing strategy helps you most. Watch for the tendency to underestimate how long it takes to do a task. If organizing proves very difficult, you may want to work with an ADHD coach or CBT therapist who can help you develop these essential skills.

FOCUS ON ONE THING AT A TIME AND KEEP COMING BACK AFTER A DISTRACTION

You're probably aware that multitasking has been shown to be less effective and more draining than focusing on one thing at a time. Mindfulness training helps us notice the urge to veer off and to self-correct before too much time goes by. The following story provides a good example.

Kirk wants to curb his multitasking habit. He chose fixing the garage door as his project. Throughout the day, he checks in to the present moment, asking himself, "What am I doing now? Is it related to the garage project?" He posted a sign in his shed with the words "GARAGE DOOR" as a cue for this practice. At one point, he caught himself standing by a pond in his yard and contemplating putting a fountain in. He deepened his awareness of the moment by taking a breath and noticing the pleasant feeling associated with a new project. He also noticed thoughts about the garage door and a feeling of annoyance that he had to go back to it. However, the moment of deeper awareness gave him an opportunity to remember his desire to change his multitasking habit. "I am going to try to stick with the garage door," he said to himself.

IF YOU MULTITASK, DO IT WITH MINDFULNESS

Sometimes, multitasking on purpose is the right thing to do. Mandy, a family therapist, has been practicing mindfulness for a while. One time she was writing her clinical notes at the end of the day and noticed herself stopping in the middle of a sentence to check her e-mail. But she had developed the awareness to see this and to "tune in" to what was going on. She noticed that in the midst of writing, she often had a feeling of boredom. The feeling would make her drop the writing and turn to her e-mail. She noted this dance with increased awareness, allowing herself to stop and check e-mail from time to time. She would also bring herself back to her writing after a short "e-mail fix." Allowing this dance, with awareness, actually helped her get through her work.

KEEP ENCOURAGING YOURSELF

Your energy and motivation are likely to wane in the middle of a task, especially if it's a long one. Come up with ways to keep yourself motivated. Review your values table or your motivation reminder, if you made one. You could also remember a time when you persevered despite a difficulty. Here's one I use for myself.

A friend of mine had the idea of hiking to the top of Half Dome in Yosemite National Park during a holiday weekend. We planned on starting out early in the morning so we could make it up and down the challenging trail in one day. I was fairly fit and thought I could do such a hike. So we drove several hours to the park, spent the night there, and then at 5 a.m. the next day, we started out. About ten minutes into it I thought to myself, "This is ridiculous. I'm so tired already. I'll never make it. I just want to turn around." While contemplating these thoughts, I saw an older man with a walking stick making his way up the trail. He was going much more slowly than we were, and with each step, he was placing his feet carefully and methodically on the ground to keep his pace. At that moment I thought, "I can do this, too. All I have to do is keep walking slowly, focusing on one step at a time. I can stop and rest when I get tired, and keep going when I'm ready. Who knows how far I'll get?" This perspective helped me to continue, enjoy the beautiful views along the way, and even go to the very top of the mountain. All along, I gave myself permission to stop, but also encouraged myself to keep going a bit more. This mindset helped me to reach my goal.

WATCH AND VARY YOUR PACE

If you're getting stuck in a task, practice doing things quickly just to get the task done. Once it's complete, you can always go over it again to check for accuracy. Try using your mindful self-coaching voice to help you along by saying "go faster" or "don't get stuck." Sometimes this works if you are obsessing or being a perfectionist.

But if you find yourself skimming when you should be paying attention to details, practice slowing down on purpose, taking several deep breaths to slow down your body and your pace. Use self-coaching to remind yourself to slow down.

TAKE BREAKS, BUT WATCH FOR THE TENDENCY TO EXTEND THEM

Take timed breaks and notice any hesitancy to return to work when your clock tells you it's time to resume. That moment is a great opportunity to notice the thoughts and feelings related to transition and working. This is also the time to activate the hate-it-but-do-it center.

LOOK FOR HELP FROM "EXTERNAL ENGINES," STRUCTURES, AND PEOPLE

Set a deadline for yourself, involve another person, or create an external structure with the use of calendars, timers, and other organizational tools that make the time dedicated to a task visible and audible. Sometimes just having someone in the room with you while you do your task (and they do something else) can make a big difference. Notice with mindfulness if this is true for you, too.

Finishing the Task

When finishing a task, try these strategies to help you be successful:

- Pay attention to closing.
- Transition out of the task.
- Forgive yourself if you drop the ball...and pick it up again.
- Reward yourself for finishing.

PAY ATTENTION TO CLOSING

Finishing or "closing" tasks is often a challenge for adults with ADHD. Check in with yourself frequently as to how you're doing as you approach the end. Do you procrastinate more or get more distracted? What body sensations, feelings, and thoughts come up when you think of finishing the job? Do you notice a sense of your energy dropping, thoughts of boredom, annoyance, or anxiety? Maybe you notice a sense of being done even if you are not really done yet? For example, you may notice the excited thought "I'm done!" when paying your bills just by having the stamped envelopes on the table with your checks enclosed. But such thoughts and feelings can later lead you to forget to put the letters in the mailbox. Note all of these observations with curiosity.

TRANSITION OUT OF THE TASK

Watch for the tendency to be stuck in hyperfocus and any difficulty transitioning from one task to another. Ask yourself, "Am I hyperfocused?" from time to time as a way to monitor your attention. Of course that can be hard to do spontaneously, so before you train yourself in the habit of checking in, write the question on a Post-it next to your work station. Use it as a cue to catch yourself hyperfocusing and enhance the awareness of what that state is like by dropping into your body awareness in that moment.

To counteract hyperfocus, you can use imagery or meditation that helps you develop a *flexible* focus. For example, imagine being a frog hopping from lily pad to lily pad with ease. Imagine that like that frog, you can hop on and off a task. See if you can sense being agile and resistant to getting stuck. Alternatively, use a hand gesture that expresses movement and flexibility for you. Use that movement to reinforce the intention for easy transition.

FORGIVE YOURSELF IF YOU DROP THE BALL . . . AND PICK IT UP AGAIN

Practice simply renewing your intention and then returning to the task, even if it is more complex now because of the delay.

REWARD YOURSELF FOR FINISHING

Notice with full awareness how it feels to be done. Pause to feel it in your body and notice your thoughts and feelings. Reward yourself, and savor the reward. This experience of mastery, enjoyment, or relief, if taken in fully with awareness, can become a great resource for you. Deepened memory of this feeling can be a great motivator later when you approach a new task.

Creating Good Habits
(Combining Mindfulness and Autopilot)

With repetitive tasks, take advantage of autopilot. First build a routine through the mindful use of your senses and repetition of the same action. Then notice the moments when you digress from the planned routine, and self-correct in the very moment you notice. Here's an example with a common problem:

Jerry keeps misplacing his keys. At least once every week he's frantically looking for them before leaving for work. He's been told that having the same spot for his keys can help the problem, so he got a decorative bowl to put them in, and he placed it on the kitchen counter. However, many times he still forgets to put the keys there and ends up missing them. So in one of our meetings we did a mindfulness exercise to help him build the desired habit.

I asked Jerry to pull out his keys and inspect them with curiosity. We started by having him notice the shapes, colors, and different metals used to make them. Then he touched the keys with his fingertips and felt for roughness, coolness, and any other sensations. He held the bunch of keys in his hand for few seconds, noting its weight. I asked him if he could practice putting them in the bowl with awareness of his intention, his arm movement, and the very act of releasing the keys from his hand. We did it several times.

When practicing at home, Jerry was to note his keys with this kind of awareness every time he handled them. He was also to say in his mind (or out loud), "I'm putting the keys in my bowl," whenever he got home, to reinforce the habit. If he noticed that he dropped the keys on the table, he was to pick them up and immediately put them in the bowl. After a while, Jerry would drop the keys in the bowl automatically without having to think about it.

EXPLORATION 8.5
Training a Good Habit

- Think of what habit you would like to strengthen. Perhaps like Jerry, you need to practice handling your keys with mindfulness. Or perhaps it is another habit, like taking vitamins in the morning or flossing at night.
- Make a point to do the action slowly and with mindfulness, noting with your senses and bringing attention to your thoughts and feelings.
- As you do the action, note in your mind what you are doing from moment to moment to strengthen your full acknowledgment of each step ("I am reaching for the floss").

MINDFULNESS FOR ADHD

- Notice, if you can, the very moment of decision to start the action and the very moment of completing it.
- If you notice yourself becoming distracted or somehow not doing the intended habit, become curious about what is stopping you and see if you can renew your intention.
- Do this for a week (or more if needed) and see if the urge to do the habit starts to arise more automatically. Use visual reminders as needed.

Time Management

Last but not least, we tackle the topic of time management. Perhaps just reading the words "time management" gives you a sinking feeling inside. If so, remember that this skill is difficult for many adults with ADHD. Trouble with planning, distractibility, forgetfulness, and impulsive decisions all contribute to this difficulty. We also know from research studies that the ability to estimate time accurately is diminished in ADHD children and adults.[3]

Adults with ADHD typically underestimate the amount of time required to complete tasks (or you could say they overestimate the amount of time they have). I often frame it as being overly optimistic when it comes to time. For example, someone with ADHD may think that going to the store will take half an hour, when in fact it takes an hour or much more.

Transition time—for example, the time it takes to leave the house when going somewhere—is often not properly factored in by adults with ADHD. I often review with my patients how long they think it takes them to get ready in the morning, then I ask them to time how long it *actually* takes them over the course of several days. Commonly they're surprised at what they find. For example, they find that an extra ten minutes passes from the moment they finish breakfast to the moment they get in the car—a lot more than they estimated. In addition, many adults with ADHD also report an urge to "do just one more thing" before they leave, which contributes to their lateness.

Another common barrier to good time management is procrastination in the form of "I'll do this when I have more time." However, the postponed tasks may never get done because more time never arrives. The saying, "There is no better time than the present" is good to remember if you tend to procrastinate in this way.

Mindfulness can help you note your thoughts and feelings related to how long an activity will take and how you handle times of transition ("This will take five minutes" or "I can fit this between my work and picking up my son"). Note your assumptions with mindfulness and later check your expectations against the actual outcome. While the way you perceive time can't be easily changed, mindful self-coaching can help. If you tend to underestimate time, develop a habit of asking yourself: "Is this a realistic estimation?" or "I need to allow time for parking there." It can also help to add an extra ten or fifteen minutes to what you *feel* is realistic.

Combine this approach with tools like a calendar and visual and audible time reminders to help you outsmart your natural assumptions about time.

Suggested Reminders for Practice

For this step, the following reminder signs can be helpful:

- Pause
- Calm Focus
- Mindful Self-Coaching

- Break It Down
- Prioritize
- Start Sideways

Step 8 at a Glance

Formal Practice

- Do fifteen minutes of mindful presence meditation each day.

Mindful Awareness in Daily Life

- Use meditation with imagery:

    - To feel calm (Mountain Meditation, or your own image).
    - To feel ready to act (tiger imagery, or your own image).
    - To have a flexible focus (frog imagery, or your own image).

- Note the *choosing — starting — doing — finishing* task sequence with mindfulness. STOP in the midst of tasks to check in and deepen awareness.

4 Putting It All Together

Using Mindfulness in Your Daily Life with ADHD

Steven owns a new gourmet cheese store. Setting up the business has been a lot of work, and he's been putting in ten-hour days. Before, he used to make time for mindful walks and quiet sitting mindfulness practice, which he says he found "very grounding." Now, however, he feels like he's busy from the moment he awakes until the moment he goes to bed at night. "I have just enough time in the evening to get dinner and talk to my girlfriend before I get really tired," he says. "My meditation practice has gone out the window."

Like Steven, we all have times when we feel like we don't have a spare moment to do anything besides eat and work. But we all need some down time to balance out even the busiest of days, and people with ADHD need this time even more. Also, some of us might need new ways to practice to keep it from becoming stale or boring, so here are some reminders for keeping mindfulness in your life:

1. If you stop practicing mindfulness for a while, renew your intention and start again. Realize you can drop into deeper awareness *anywhere, anytime,* even if it's only for a moment or two. Connect with the present by noticing

your breath in the very moment you happened to think of mindfulness.

2. Use visual or electronic reminders to practice awareness of the present moment. If a reminder becomes so familiar that you tend to ignore it, come up with a new one.

3. In your calendar, schedule times for quiet sitting, mindful movement, or even a mindful day. You can sign up for a daylong retreat through your local meditation center or design one on your own.

4. Schedule and use time in nature as a simple mindfulness practice. Notice plants and hear sounds around you with curiosity. Notice your body and check in with how you feel when, for example, walking, hiking, cycling, or simply sitting in a park.

5. Sign up for a mindfulness meditation class to renew your interest in and understanding of mindfulness. The class structure and support of the teacher and fellow participants can help you stay consistent. Alternatively, join an online mindfulness community and get e-mail reminders, quotes, and suggestions for practice. Try, for example, www.eMindful.com.

6. Find a mindfulness buddy—someone who's exploring mindfulness, too. Help each other keep practicing mindfulness.

7. Go to talks on mindfulness, read a book, or listen to a CD on the topic. Even if you're slow to do the practice, the reading can help you make the shift to be more present in daily life.

8. Keep a mindfulness journal or a scrapbook and use it to reflect on moments of presence and awareness in your life.

9. Sign up for an improvisation class or do yoga, tai chi, dance, rock climbing, or other exercises with the intention to be more present to your body, your thoughts, and feelings.

10. Remind yourself to be mindful in everyday places, such as when shopping, driving, or watching TV. Let every

moment be an opportunity for a deeper connection with yourself and your life.

Going through Your Typical Day with Mindful Awareness On

Weave mindfulness into your daily routine. In the morning, instead of jolting out of bed, try noticing the sensations of your body as you get up or stretch. Right then set the intention to be more aware throughout the day, knowing you can always pause and check in with your attention and the present moment.

Use elements of your morning routine as opportunities for training attention and awareness. For example, in the shower, notice the tendency to quickly go on autopilot and become lost in thinking. Then see if you can use the shower as a practice period where you bring attention to your senses — smelling the soap, feeling the sensation of the water on your body, listening to the sounds that are present. You can also bring attention to your senses as you eat your breakfast, noting the smell, warmth, and taste of coffee or your food. If you have an exercise routine, note with curiosity your movements, breathing, and body sensations as you work out.

When getting ready to leave the house, notice if your intention to be on time matches your preparations from moment to moment. Do you get sidetracked or try to pack in too many last-minute things before you go? As you bring nonjudgmental awareness to these ADHD patterns, also notice how it feels to let go of the distractions and diversions. With increased awareness you'll have more ability to pull yourself away from unhelpful patterns.

As you leave the house, notice the tendency to rush and tense your body. Instead, take a deep breath and soften your body. Bring attention to your keys, and, with increased awareness, pick them up and place them in your bag or your pocket. Then slow down slightly as you walk to the car, and try to remain relaxed as you drive. If you're running late, see if you can note and label what's happening: for example, "being late," "feeling frazzled," or "an urge to speed." Then practice accepting that, without being overly reactive or speeding. As you drive, let red lights be reminders to notice your breath.

In conversations, bring attention to your talking style. Check for an urge to interrupt, include too much information, or veer off the main topic. Become curious about any other automatic patterns—for example, a knee-jerk reaction to automatically agree or disagree with the other person. With increased awareness of your communication style you will have more choice in directing your message. Practice mindful listening and talking with your loved ones.

When doing tasks at work, bring curiosity to the process of starting and finishing them. Notice how you work, and check for feelings of reluctance to stay with or complete something. Notice the effort needed to finally close a task. Be curious about what thoughts and feelings are present throughout this process.

Through the day, periodically check in to see if you're feeling overwhelmed, or whether you feel on top of things. Are you feeling paralyzed, or motivated and energized? Maybe you notice a tendency to procrastinate on an important or a complex task. Try to bring nonjudgmental awareness to what's happening, and use STOP or RAIN reminders to check more deeply into your body, thoughts, feelings, and actions. If you're feeling overwhelmed, take some time to connect with the breath and allow your body to relax—things may look different after that. Or you may find that once you label what's happening—for example, "procrastination," "fear," or "doubting"—you can step back from the experience and no longer identify with it. You're also creating an opening to renew the intention and the effort to tackle the task one step at a time.

As you interact with coworkers and others, try to bring more attention, presence, and a nonjudgmental attitude. See if you can be curious about both the uniqueness as well as the common qualities of yourself and other people.

When you take a break from work or your daily routine, explore different ways of visually attending to an object. For example, when looking at a picture, focus on the most obvious element of the picture. Then focus on the background. Try opening your awareness to both at the same time.

When you're done with work, check in to and relax your body when making your way back home. As you enter your home, bring awareness to that moment—for instance, setting down your keys and where you place them. Ideally pick one place and practice putting or returning keys to that spot with full awareness.

Once you're home, greet your loved ones with full attention and presence for them. Express love, concern, and compassion in your interactions. Feel and express gratitude for who they are and what they do. Be a mindful presence, for yourself and others.

Mindfulness for the Kid in Your Family (and the Kid in You)

Kathy's eight-year-old son, Warren, has ADHD. Kathy has been learning about mindfulness and thinks the approach has helped her become less stressed, more focused, and connected to her life in a new way. She has been more present to Warren in their interactions and enjoys their time together in a fuller way. Learning about ADHD as well as mindfulness has helped her understand her son's difficulties with more compassion and increased resilience. When we talk, she says, "I wish Warren could learn this. He is so high-strung and gets upset easily. Are there any resources to teach kids mindfulness?"

Imagine a group of five- to six-year-olds lying in a circle in the middle of their classroom floor. Their mindfulness teacher softly instructs them: "Put the bear on your belly and watch it coming up and down." Each child now has a tiny stuffed bear bobbing to the rhythm of their breathing. As they watch their breath, the typically fidgety bunch slowly calms down. This mindfulness technique is used by Susan Kaiser Greenland, the founder of the Innerkids foundation, an organization that teaches kids mindful awareness. Similar playful exercises get the kids to watch their mind and balance their emotions. The kids also learn how to be more compassionate and more connected with each other.

This type of education is sorely needed today, when so many kids can feel stressed or isolated. As Innerkids and other organizations are introducing mindfulness to young children, there's a growing excitement about giving children such basic skills that are often overlooked in today's school curriculum.[1]

Adults with ADHD who like to learn in a visual and kinesthetic way may find mindfulness exercises for kids informative and easier to grasp. And if you're a parent, the exercises are something fun and useful you can do together with your child. You may even find that the kids will end up teaching you. For more on mindfulness for kids, see Susan Kaiser Greenland's book, *The Mindful Child*, as well as other similar books.

A Note on Psychology, Mindfulness, and Spirituality

In this book I present mindfulness primarily as a psychological approach and focus on it as a mind state that can be helpful in developing awareness and self-regulation in coping with ADHD. But it's important to realize that the mindfulness tradition is more than a psychological technique—it's also an ethical and spiritual path. Concepts of the impermanence of self and reality, overcoming ego-driven desire, and the interdependence of all living things are important mindfulness teachings. The path of mindfulness teaches morality and develops compassion toward self and others, even one's enemies.

I believe that studying and living out these concepts, whether through secular mindfulness programs or through the Buddhist or other spiritual traditions, are ways to deepen psychological healing and wholeness. Overall, it can be said that the psychological approach focuses on integrating the self, while mindfulness and the spiritual path focus on transcending the self. Together—psychology, mindfulness, and spirituality—they can complement each other and promote personal growth and resilience.

Closing Remarks: Living With and Loving Your ADHD Life

Our lives happen as a string of present moments that are constantly arising and passing. How we meet such moments makes an immense difference in the unfolding of our life. Mindfulness—awareness of the present moment with curiosity and kindness—helps us "show up" in our life, however it is. Without such awareness we can end up merely going through the motions, feeling stressed and unhappy, and missing the full potential in ourselves and others.

And what if the life we have is a life with ADHD? Often life with ADHD is a dance of discouragement and hope, where moments of play, joy, or accomplishment can be followed by moments of doubt, fear, or despair. Knowing that we can always access the space of mindful awareness—awareness that can hold any experience with openness and compassion—can be a lifeline. That's because this knowing is also a realization that freedom and healing is possible, even if a complete cure is not. Mindfulness is a resource that brings resilience and hope. It can sustain and surprise us in endless ways, moment by moment.

Mindfulness practice involves love, trust, and courage. It is an act of love to decide that your inner experience matters and deserves your full attention. It is an act of trust that even in the midst of failure or struggle there is always more right with you than wrong with you, ADHD or not. It is an act of courage to let awareness hold everything—even the greatest pain—even if you don't think that you can hold it. With mindfulness at your side, you can welcome your ADHD life and everything it brings with acceptance and deep appreciation for the ADHD moments—and all the other moments in between.

Ultimately, mindfulness gives us a profound awareness that there is beauty and mystery in us that is beyond all labels or stories we have about ourselves and others. We grow to know deeply that no matter what our thoughts or feelings are doing in that moment, there is also an inner resource that can answer with insight and kindness. We learn to observe and discern with wisdom. We also grow to know that as we struggle with our imperfections we are nevertheless whole—even in ADHD moments, even in this very moment.

Thank you for taking the time to read this book and being open to exploring this new way of being present with yourself, your ADHD, and the rest of your life. I hope that you will find this approach as helpful as I have, empowering, and healing. And most of all, I hope that you will make it your own.

Frequently Asked Questions (FAQ)

Q: Should I try medication or meditation?

The answer depends on several things—mainly how bad your ADHD symptoms are and how motivated you are to try something other than medication. I usually recommend trying both. Medication works well for many people, and it may make a big difference for you. In fact, medications may enhance your ability for mindfulness, especially the ability to pause, withhold an impulse, and self-reflect. However, if you experience significant side effects—or want to minimize relying on medications—you should investigate the nonpharmaceutical approaches such as cognitive-behavioral therapy or meditation. Some people, especially those with milder symptoms, can do fine with only nonpharmaceutical approaches.

Just as with other cognitive trainings, it's likely that a skill such as mindfulness can complement medications so they can either be lowered or they can be kept at the same level but with a resulting improvement in ADHD symptoms. However, at this point, research specifically on the relationship of medications and meditation in ADHD is yet to be done.

Q: Will ADHD medications interfere with my mindfulness practice, or will they perhaps help it?

Try it and see! When it comes to the sitting meditation practice, I know that some people have found that taking an ADHD medication helped them focus and curb their restlessness during their sitting session. Others found that the medication made them impatient to do tasks, and they preferred to do the sitting practice without their medications. As mentioned above, some patients report that stimulant medications make them more naturally reflective or mindful in daily life. Others felt more driven and engrossed in doing whatever task they were working on. Whatever you choose to do, you can still use mindful awareness to observe the result on your practice and your daily actions.

Q: I thought meditation, including mindfulness, is a type of spiritual practice. Is that true? And if so, what if I already have a spiritual practice?

It's true that in Buddhist, Hindu, Islamic, Christian, or Jewish religions, meditation is often a spiritual practice. At the same time, mindfulness can be used as a secular tool to enhance physical and psychological functioning and to promote brain health. Mindfulness meditation is now taught in clinics and hospitals in a secular way (for example, at the UCLA Mindful Awareness Research Center). When practicing mindfulness in this way, you don't have to adopt any specific spiritual outlook.

However, even in secular courses on mindfulness, ethics are often discussed along with topics such as friendliness, compassion, forgiveness, and gratefulness. Such universal teachings support the practice of mindfulness and can be related to your own spiritual practice, no matter what it is.

Q: In meditation, your mind is supposed to go blank. Mine never stops.

There are many misconceptions about how meditation is supposed to be, and this is one of them.

When you first start mindfulness exercises, you'll often notice how busy your mind is. With more practice, or with more intense relaxation, you may experience some quieting of the mind—but that's not necessary to have a successful mindfulness experience. Successful practice is being aware of the present moment no matter how it is.

Q: Do I have to do sitting meditation to learn mindfulness?

No, you don't. You can practice mindful moments in your daily life and still learn and benefit from it. For example, if you're having intense emotions during the course of your day, you can practice mindful awareness while in the midst of the experience, by noting the feelings in your body and practicing self-compassion (discussed in step 6). Practices such as yoga, tai chi, and martial arts, when done with a focus on awareness, can also be good ways to train present-moment focus.

Q: Why even bother with sitting meditation?

Sitting meditation provides an opportunity to observe your experience in silence and with "non-doing"—in contrast to much of our daily lives. This helps us see subtle shifts of awareness or notice things we wouldn't otherwise have noticed. It creates a "laboratory" for training your attention and expanding your insight, and helps you experience yourself in a new way. For that reason I recommend doing sitting meditation at least sometimes, either at home or by signing up for a class or workshop. Even if you find it difficult to keep up with sitting meditation regularly in your daily life, the experience may prove very informative, even transforming.

Q: To be mindful, I am supposed to be nonjudgmental. Does that mean I don't make any judgments, or "anything goes"?

In everyday life we sometimes use the words "judging" and "judgmental" to describe someone as being overly critical or condemning. However, judgment also means discernment, good judgment, and knowing right from wrong. Sometimes those starting to practice mindfulness worry that you're not supposed to make any judgments, even good ones. So it's important to clarify this point.

In mindfulness, the nonjudgmental stance is the first step on the road to developing a healthy relationship with yourself and overall good judgment. In mindful self-observation, by initially suspending any judgment, we create the openness to see everything with clarity and without preconceived notions such as "this is good" or "this is bad." This nonjudgmental stance allows us to notice our thoughts and feelings in a non-reactive way.

This initial stance allows for full acceptance of what is and expands awareness of what is involved. In the process, our beliefs can be fully examined. In this way, mindfulness paves the way for sound judgment to arise in daily life, and if needed, facilitates a healthy change. The nonjudgmental observation, especially when combined with ethics, supports discernment of what's helpful and what isn't, what's moral and what's immoral. In this way, mindfulness and good judgment go hand in hand.

ADHD Symptoms Checklist

Patient Name	Today's Date

Please answer the questions below, rating yourself on each of the criteria shown using the scale on the right side of the page. As you answer each question, place an X in the box that best describes how you have felt and conducted yourself over the past 6 months.

	Never	Rarely	Sometimes	Often	Very Often
1. How often do you have trouble wrapping up the final details of a project, once the challenging parts have been done?					
2. How often do you have difficulty getting things in order when you have to do a task that requires organization?					
3. How often do you have problems remembering appointments or obligations?					
4. When you have a task that requires a lot of thought, how often do you avoid or delay getting started?					
5. How often do you fidget or squirm with your hands or feet when you have to sit down for a long time?					
6. How often do you feel overly active and compelled to do things, like you were driven by a motor?					
Part A					
7. How often do you make careless mistakes when you have to work on a boring or difficult project?					
8. How often do you have difficulty keeping your attention when you are doing boring or repetitive work?					

9. How often do you have difficulty concentrating on what people say to you, even when they are speaking to you directly?					
10. How often do you misplace or have difficulty finding things at home or at work?					
11. How often are you distracted by activity or noise around you?					
12. How often do you leave your seat in meetings or other situations in which you are expected to remain seated?					
13. How often do you feel restless or fidgety?					
14. How often do you have difficulty unwinding and relaxing when you have time to yourself?					
15. How often do you find yourself talking too much when you are in social situations?					
16. When you're in a conversation, how often do you find yourself finishing the sentences of the people you are talking to, before they can finish them themselves?					
17. How often do you have difficulty waiting your turn in situations when turn taking is required?					
18. How often do you interrupt others when they are busy?					

Part B

Questions from the World Health Organization Adult ADHD Self-Report Scale (ASRS-v1.1) Symptom Checklist. You can download a printable version of this table from www.shambhala.com/MindfulnessPrescription.

Instructions

Symptoms

1. Complete both parts A and B of the symptom checklist[1] by marking an X in the box that most closely represents the frequency of occurrence of each of the symptoms.
2. Score part A. If four or more marks appear in the darkly shaded boxes within part A then you have symptoms highly consistent with ADHD in adults and further investigation is warranted.
3. The frequency scores on part B provide additional cues and can serve as further probes into the your symptoms. Pay particular attention to marks appearing in the dark shaded boxes.

Functional Impairments

1. Evaluate the level of impairment associated with your symptom.
2. Consider work, school, social, and family settings.
3. Think of how these problems have affected your ability to work, take care of things at home, or get along with other people such as your spouse or significant other.

Childhood History

Assess the presence of these symptoms or similar symptoms in childhood. You need not have been formally diagnosed as a child but look for evidence of early and persistent problems with your attention or self-control. Some significant symptoms should have been present in childhood, but full set of symptoms is not necessary.

Key

Questions representing inattentive symptoms: 1, 2, 3, 4, 7, 8, 9, 10, 11

Questions representing hyperactive or impulsive symptoms: 5, 6, 11, 12, 13, 14, 15, 16, 17, 18

List of Mindfulness Exercises

STEP 1

Exploration 1.1: Playing with Visual Attention and Awareness

Exploration 1.2: Playing with Non-Visual Attention

Exploration 1.3: Tuning In to the Five Senses

Exploration 1.4: Mindful Eating

STEP 2

Exploration 2.1: Noting the Breath in Three Places

Exploration 2.2: Mindful Breathing (CD track 2)

Exploration 2.3: Mindful Breathing and Walking

STEP 3

Exploration 3.1: Listening to Music

Exploration 3.2: Mindfulness of Sound, Breath and Body (CD track 3)

Exploration 3.3: The STOP Practice

STEP 4

Exploration 4.1: Body Scan (CD track 4)

Exploration 4.2: Mindful Movement

Exploration 4.3: Mindful Walking (CD track 5)

Exploration 4.4: Shaking and Dancing Meditation

Exploration 4.5: Working with Restlessness

STEP 5

Exploration 5.1: Mind Like a Sky (CD track 6)

Exploration 5.2: Watching Your Thinking under a Tree

Exploration 5.3: Mind Like an Ocean

STEP 6

Exploration 6.1: Pleasant, Unpleasant, and Neutral Events

Exploration 6.2: RAIN (CD track 7)

Exploration 6.3: Loving-Kindness Meditation (CD track 8)

STEP 7

Exploration 7.1: STOP as You Talk

Exploration 7.2: Mindful Listening and Speaking

Exploration 7.3: Mindful Presence (CD track 9)

STEP 8

Exploration 8.1: Using the STOP Practice with Tasks

Exploration 8.2: The Mountain Meditation

Exploration 8.3: Values Worksheet

Exploration 8.4: "Breathing In, I Am Like..."

Exploration 8.5: Training a Good Habit

Notes

Dear Reader: Do Something Different This Time

1. Jeffrey M. Greeson, "Mindfulness Research Update: 2008," *Complementary Health Practice Review* 14, no. 1 (January 2009): 10–18; and Lisa Flook et al., "Effects of Mindful Awareness Practices on Executive Functions in Elementary School Children," *Journal of Applied School Psychology* 26, no. 1 (2010): 70–95.
2. See Britta Hölzel et al., "Mindfulness Practice Leads to Increases in Regional Brain Gray Matter Density," *Psychiatry Research* 191, no. 1 (2011): 36–43; and Antoine Lutz et al., "Mental Training Enhances Attentional Stability: Neural and Behavioral Evidence," *Journal of Neuroscience* 29, no. 42 (October 2009): 13418–13427.
3. Lidia Zylowska et al., "Mindfulness Meditation Training in Adults and Adolescents with Attention Deficit Hyperactivity Disorder: A Feasibility Study," *Journal of Attention Disorders* 11, no. 6 (May 2008): 737–746.

Chapter 1. A Different Way of Paying Attention

1. Jefferey N. Epstein and Yehoshua Tsal, "Evidence for Cognitive Training as a Treatment Strategy for Children with Attention-Deficit/Hyperactivity Disorder," *Journal of ADHD and Related Disorders* 1 no. 2 (2010): 49–64.
2. Kirk Warren Brown, Richard M. Ryan, and J. David Creswell, "Mindfulness: Theoretical Foundations and Evidence for Its Salutary Effects," *Psychological Inquiry* 18, no. 4 (2007): 211–237.
3. See Lidia Zylowska, Susan Smalley, and Jeffrey Schwartz, "Mindfulness for Attention Deficit Hyperactivity Disorder," in *Clinical*

Handbook of Mindfulness, ed. Fabrizio Didona (New York: Springer-Verlag, 2008); and Shruti Baijal and Rashmi Gupta, "Meditation-Based Training: A Possible Intervention for Attention Deficit Hyperactivity Disorder," *Psychiatry* 5, no. 4 (April 2008): 48–55.

4. Zindel V. Segal, J. Mark G. Williams, and John D. Teasdale, *Mindfulness-Based Cognitive Therapy for Depression: A New Approach to Preventing Relapse* (New York: Guilford, 2002).

5. Scott R. Bishop et al., "Mindfulness: A Proposed Operational Definition," *Clinical Psychology Science and Practice* 11, no. 3 (2004): 230–241.

6. Ruth A. Baer et al., "Construct Validity of the Five Facet Mindfulness Questionnaire in Meditating and Nonmeditating Samples," *Assessment* 15, no. 3 (2008): 329–342.

7. Jon Kabat-Zinn, *Full Catastrophe Living: Using the Wisdom of Your Body and Mind to Face Stress, Pain, and Illness* (New York: Delacorte Press, 1990).

8. See Segal, Williams, and Teasdale.

9. For discussion of Dialectical Behavioral Therapy (DBT) and Acceptance Commitment Therapy (ACT), see Steven C. Hayes, Victoria M. Follette, and Marsha M. Linehan, eds., *Mindfulness and Acceptance: Expanding the Cognitive-Behavioral Tradition* (New York: Guilford, 2004). For mindfulness in Gestalt therapy, see Philip Brownell, *Gestalt Therapy: A Guide to Contemporary Practice* (New York: Springer, 2010).

10. Alberto Chiesa, Raffaella Calati, and Alessandro Serretti, "Does Mindfulness Training Improve Cognitive Abilities? A Systematic Review of Neuropsychological Findings," *Clinical Psychology Review* 31, no. 3 (April 2011): 449–464.

11. Melissa A. Tanner et al., "The Effects of The Transcendental Meditation Program on Mindfulness," *Journal of Clinical Psychology* (2009): 574–589.

12. Susan L. Smalley et al., "Mindfulness and Attention Deficit Hyperactivity Disorder," *Journal of Clinical Psychology* 65, no. 1 (2009): 1087–1098.

Chapter 2. Mindfulness and Self-Regulation in ADHD

1. Walter Mischel, Yuichi Shoda, and Monica L. Rodriguez, "Delay of Gratification in Children," *Science* n.s. 244, no. 4907 (May 1989): 933–938.

2. Jonah Lehrer, "Don't! The Secret of Self-Control," *New Yorker,* 18 May 2009, 26–32.

3. Russell A. Barkley, *ADHD and the Nature of Self-Control* (New York: Guilford, 1997). The 2006 paperback edition has a new afterword.

4. Russell A. Barkley, "The Nature of ADHD: The Executive Functions and Self Regulation," lecture at the 2010 CHADD Conference in Atlanta, GA, presented November 11, 2010.

5. Brandon J. Schmeichel and Roy F. Baumeister, "Self-Regulatory Strength," in Baumeister and Kathleen Vohs, eds., *Handbook of Self-Regulation*, 2nd ed. (New York: Guilford Press, 2011), 64–82.

6. Barkley, *ADHD and the Nature of Self-Control*.

7. Russell A. Barkley, *Taking Charge of Adult ADHD* (New York: Guilford Press, 2010).

8. See Lidia Zylowska, Susan Smalley, and Jeffrey Schwartz, "Mindfulness for Attention Deficit Hyperactivity Disorder," in *Clinical Handbook of Mindfulness*, ed. Fabrizio Didona (New York: Springer-Verlag, 2008); and Shruti Baijal and Rashmi Gupta, "Meditation-Based Training: A Possible Intervention for Attention Deficit Hyperactivity Disorder," *Psychiatry* 5, no. 4 (April 2008): 48–55.

9. Bernd Hesslinger et al., "Psychotherapy of Attention Deficit Hyperactivity Disorder in Adults: A Pilot Study Using a Structured Skills Training Program," *European Archives of Psychiatry and Clinical Neuroscience* 252, no. 4 (2002): 177–184; and Alexandra Philipsen et al., "Structured Group Psychotherapy in Adults with Attention Deficit Hyperactivity Disorder: Results of an Open Multicentre Study," *Journal of Nervous and Mental Disease* 195, no. 12 (2007): 1013–1019.

10. Philipsen et al., 1013–1019.

11. Nirbhay N. Singh et al., "Mindfulness Training for Parents and Their Children with ADHD Increases the Children's Compliance," *Journal of Child and Family Studies* 19, no. 2 (2010): 157–166.

12. Saskia van der Oord, Susan M. Bögels, and Dorreke Peijnenburg, "The Effectiveness of Mindfulness Training for Children with ADHD and Mindful Parenting for their Parents," *Journal of Child Family Studies* (February 2011): 1–9.

13. Linda J. Harrison, Ramesh Manocha, and Katya Rubia, "Sahaja Yoga Meditation as Family Treatment Programme for Children with Attention Deficit Hyperactivity Disorder," *Clinical Child Psychology and Psychiatry* 9, no. 4 (2004): 479–497.

14. Sarina J. Grosswald et al., "Use of the Transcendental Meditation Technique to Reduce Symptoms of Attention Deficit Hyperactivity Disorder (ADHD) by Reducing Stress and Anxiety: An Exploratory Study," *Current Issues in Education* 10, no. 2 (December 2008), http://cie.asu.edu/volume10/number2/.

15. Peng Pang, "Alternative Treatment for Teenagers with Mental Illness: Results from a Twelve-Week Controlled Pilot Study," American Psychiatric Association 2010 Annual Meeting, abstract

NR2-77, presented 24 May 2010; and Maria Hernandez-Reif, Tiffany Field, and Eric Thimas, "Adolescents with Attention Deficit Hyperactivity Disorder Benefit from Tai Chi," *Journal of Bodywork and Movement Therapies* 5, no. 2 (2001): 120–123.

16. Amishi P. Jha, Jason Krompinger, and Michael J. Baime, "Mindfulness Training Modifies Subsystems of Attention," *Cognitive, Affective, & Behavioral Neuroscience* 7, no. 2 (2007): 109–119.

17. Katherine A. MacLean et al., "Intensive Meditation Training Improves Perceptual Discrimination and Sustained Attention," *Psychological Science* 21, no. 6 (2010): 829–839.

18. Alberto Chiesa, Raffaella Calati, and Alessandro Serretti, "Does Mindfulness Training Improve Cognitive Abilities? A Systematic Review of Neuropsychological Findings," *Clinical Psychology Review* 31, no. 3 (April 2011): 449–464.

19. Richard Chambers, Barbara Chuen Yee Lo, and Nicholas B. Allen, "The Impact of Intensive Mindfulness Training on Attentional Control, Cognitive Style, and Affect," *Cognitive Therapy and Research* 32, no. 3 (2008): 303–322.

20. Amishi P. Jha et al., "Examining the Protective Effects of Mindfulness Training on Working Memory Capacity and Affective Experience," *Emotion* 10, no. 1 (2010): 54–64.

21. Lisa Flook et al., "Effects of Mindful Awareness Practices on Executive Functions in Elementary School Children," *Journal of Applied School Psychology* 26, no. 1 (2010): 70–95.

22. Russell A. Barkley and Mariellen Fischer, "The Unique Contribution of Emotional Impulsiveness to Impairment in Major Life Activities in Hyperactive Children as Adults," *Journal of the American Academy of Child and Adolescent Psychiatry* 49, no. 5 (May 2010): 503–513.

23. Richard Chambers, Eleonora Gullone, and Nicholas B. Allen, "Mindful Emotion Regulation: An Integrative Review," *Clinical Psychology Review* 29 (2009): 560–572.

24. John D. Teasdale et al., "Prevention of Relapse/Recurrence in Major Depression by Mindfulness-Based Cognitive Therapy," *Journal of Consulting and Clinical Psychology* 68, no. 4 (2000): 615–623.

25. Willem Kuyken et al., "Mindfulness-Based Cognitive Therapy to Prevent Relapse in Recurrent Depression," *Journal of Consulting and Clinical Psychology* 76 (2008): 966–978.

26. Kirk Warren Brown and Richard M. Ryan, "The Benefits of Being Present: Mindfulness and Its Role in Psychological Well-Being," *Journal of Personality and Social Psychology* 84, no. 4 (2003): 822–848.

27. Nirbhay N. Singh et al., "Individuals with Mental Illness Can Control Their Aggressive Behavior through Mindfulness Training," *Behavior Modification* 31, no. 3 (May 2007): 313–328.

28. Jeffrey M. Greeson, "Mindfulness Research Update: 2008," *Complementary Health Practice Review* 14, no. 1 (January 2009): 10–18.

29. Rodrigo Escobar et al., "Worse Quality of Life for Children with Newly Diagnosed Attention-Deficit/Hyperactivity Disorder, Compared with Asthmatic and Healthy Children," *Pediatrics* 116, no. 3 (September 2005): 364–369.

30. Val A. Harpin, "The Effect of ADHD on the Life of an Individual, Their Family, and Community from Preschool to Adult Life," *Archives of Disease in Childhood* 90, suppl. 1 (February 2005): i2–i7.

31. See the Mindfulness Research Guide at www.mindfulexperience.org/publications.php.

32. Richard J. Davidson et al., "Alterations in Brain and Immune Function Produced by Mindfulness Meditation," *Psychosomatic Medicine* 65, no. 4 (2003): 564–570.

33. See Harpin and Laurel Eakin, et al., "The Marital and Family Functioning of Adults with ADHD and Their Spouses," in *Journal of Attention Disorders* 8 no 1 (2004): 1–10.

34. David W. Goodman, "The Consequences of Attention-Deficit/Hyperactivity Disorder in Adults," *Journal of Psychiatric Practice* 13, no. 5 (2007): 318–327.

35. Daniel J. Siegel, *The Mindful Brain: Reflection and Attunement in the Cultivation of Well-Being* (New York: Norton, 2007).

36. James W. Carson et al., "Mindfulness-Based Relationship Enhancement," *Behavior Therapy* 35, no. 3 (2004): 471–494.

37. Ludwig Grepmair et al., "Promoting Mindfulness in Psychotherapists in Training Influences the Treatment Results of Their Patients: A Randomized, Double-Blind, Controlled Study," *Psychotherapy and Psychosomatics* 76, no. 6 (2007): 332–338.

38. See Sharon Begley, *Train Your Mind, Change Your Brain: How a New Science Reveals Our Extraordinary Potential to Transform Ourselves* (New York: Ballantine Books, 2007); and Jeffrey M. Schwartz and Sharon Begley, *The Mind and the Brain: Neuroplasticity and the Power of Mental Force* (New York: HarperCollins, 2002).

39. Eleanor A. Maguire, Katherine Woollett, and Hugo J. Spiers. "London Taxi Drivers and Bus Drivers: A Structural MRI and Neuropsychological Analysis," *Hippocampus* 16 (2006): 1091–1101.

40. Torkel Klingberg et al., "Computerized Training of Working Memory in Children with ADHD: A Randomized, Controlled Trial," *Journal of the American Academy of Child and Adolescent Psychiatry* 44, no. 2 (2005): 177–186.

41. Gregg H. Recanzone, Christoph E. Schreiner, and Michael M. Merzenich, "Plasticity in the Frequency Representation of

Primary Auditory Cortex following Discrimination Training in Adult Owl Monkeys," *Journal of Neuroscience* 13, no. 1 (January 1993): 87–103.

42. Sara W. Lazar et al., "Meditation Experience Is Associated with Increased Cortical Thickness," *Neuroreport* 16, no. 17 (2005): 1893–1897.

43. Heleen A. Slagter et al., "Mental Training Affects Distribution of Limited Brain Resources," *PLoS Biology* 5, no. 6 (June 2007): e138.

44. Yi-Yuan Tang et al., "Short-Term Meditation Training Improves Attention and Self-Regulation," *PNAS* 104, no. 43 (2007): 17152–17156.

45. Britta Hölzel et al., "Mindfulness Practice Leads to Increases in Regional Brain Gray Matter Density," *Psychiatry Research* 191, no. 1 (January 2011): 36–43.

Chapter 3. Getting Ready for the Eight-Step Program

1. J. David Creswell et al., "Neural Correlates of Disposition Mindfulness during Affect Labeling," *Psychosomatic Medicine* 69, no. 6 (2007): 560–565.

Step 1. Become More Present

1. Michael Posner et al., "Analyzing and Shaping Human Attentional Networks," *Neural Networks* 19, no. 9 (November 2006): 1422–1429.

2. Jennifer C. Mullane et al., "Alerting, Orienting, and Executive Attention in Children with ADHD," *Journal of Attention Disorders* 15, no. 4 (May 2011): 310–320.

3. Named after the Danish psychologist Edgar Rubin, who first presented this optical illusion in his 1915 study *Synsoplevede Figurer* (Visual Figures).

4. I am indebted to the psychologist and neurofeedback pioneer Dr. Les Fehmi for emphasizing the *awareness of space, timelessness, nothingness, or absence* in facilitation of an open-awareness state. Dr. Fehmi has described an approach similar to mindfulness derived from his work with neurofeedback. His book *Open-Focus Brain: Harnessing the Power of Attention to Heal Mind and Body* (with Jim Robbins; Boston: Trumpeter, 2007) describes practices such as looking at a painting, noticing its foreground, expanding the focus to simultaneously include its background, then expanding the focus further to include the awareness of space between yourself and the painting.

5. The raisin exercise was first described in Jon Kabat-Zinn, *Full Catastrophe Living: Using the Wisdom of Your Body and Mind to Face Stress, Pain, and Illness* (New York: Delacorte Press, 1990).

Step 3. Direct and Anchor Your Awareness

1. Devarajan Sridharan et al., "Neural Dynamics of Event Segmentation in Music: Converging Evidence for Dissociable Ventral and Dorsal Streams," *Neuron* 55, no. 3 (August 2007): 521–532.

Step 4. Listen to Your Body

1. The body-scan exercise is modeled after one described in Jon Kabat-Zinn, *Full Catastrophe Living: Using the Wisdom of Your Body and Mind to Face Stress, Pain, and Illness* (New York: Delacorte Press, 1990).
2. Ellen Fliers et al., "Motor Coordination Problems in Children and Adolescents with ADHD Rated by Parents and Teachers: Effects of Age and Gender," *Journal of Neural Transmission* 115, no. 2 (2008): 11–20.
3. Mariya V. Cherkasova and Lily Hechtman, "Neuroimaging in Attention-Deficit Hyperactivity Disorder: Beyond the Frontostriatal Circuitry," *Canadian Journal of Psychiatry* 54, no. 10 (October 2009): 651–664.
4. Dana R. Carney, Amy J. C. Cuddy, and Andy J. Yap, "Power Posing: Brief Nonverbal Displays Affect Neuroendocrine Levels and Risk Tolerance," *Psychological Science* 21, no. 10 (October 2010): 1363–1368.
5. James Gordon, *Unstuck: Your Guide to the Seven-Stage Journey Out of Depression* (New York: Penguin, 2008).

Step 5. Observe Your Mind

1. Julie Sarno Owens et al., "A Critical Review of Self-Perceptions and the Positive Illusory Bias in Children with ADHD," *Clinical Child and Family Psychology Review* 10, no. 4 (2007): 335–351.
2. Nicole M. Evangelista et al., "The Positive Illusory Bias: Do Inflated Self-Perceptions in Children with ADHD Generalize to Perceptions of Others?" *Journal of Abnormal Child Psychology* 36, no. 5 (July 2008): 779–791.
3. Laura E. Knouse et al., "Accuracy of Self-Evaluation in Adults with ADHD: Evidence from a Driving Study," *Journal of Attention Disorders* 8, no. 4 (May 2005): 221–234.
4. Catherine M. Golden, "The Positive Illusory Bias: An Examination of Self-Perceptions in Adults with ADHD Symptomatology"

(master's thesis, Ohio University, 2007), http://etd.ohiolink.edu/ send-pdf.cgi/Golden%20Catherine%20M.pdf?ohiou1169218713.

5. Norman A. S. Farb et al., "Attending to the Present: Mindfulness Meditation Reveals Distinct Neural Modes of Self-Reference," *Social Cognitive and Affective Neuroscience* 2, no. 4 (2007): 313–322.

6. Ed Watkins and John D. Teasdale, "Rumination and Overgeneral Memory in Depression: Effects of Self-Focus and Analytic Thinking," *Journal of Abnormal Psychology* 110, no. 2 (May 2001): 353–357.

7. Richard J. Davidson, "Well-Being and Affective Style: Neural Substrates and Biobehavioural Correlates," *Philosophical Transactions of the Royal Society* 359 (2004): 1395–1411.

8. See Kalina Christoff, Alan Gordon, and Rachell Smith, "The Role of Spontaneous Thought in Human Cognition," in *Neuroscience of Decision Making,* eds. Oshin Vartanian and David R. Mandel (London: Psychology Press, 2011); and Kalina Christoff et al., "Experience Sampling during fMRI Reveals Default Network and Executive System Contributions to Mind Wandering," *Proceedings of the National Academy of Sciences* 106, no. 21 (2009): 8719–8724.

9. See Kalina Christoff et al. (2009), pp. 8719–8724.

10. Jonathan W. Schooler, "Re-representing Consciousness: Dissociations between Experience and Meta-Consciousness." *Trends in Cognitive Sciences* 6, no. 8 (August 2002): 339–344, and personal communication, September 24, 2010.

11. Marsha M. Linehan, *Skills Training Manual for Treating Borderline Personality Disorder* (New York: Guilford, 1993).

12. Bernd Hesslinger et al., "Psychotherapy of Attention Deficit Hyperactivity Disorder in Adults: A Pilot Study Using a Structured Skills Training Program," *European Archives of Psychiatry and Clinical Neuroscience* 252, no. 4 (2002): 177–184.

13. http://en.wikipedia.org/wiki/Serenity_Prayer. Accessed October 1, 2010.

14. Steven A. Safren et al., *Mastering Your Adult ADHD: A Cognitive-Behavioral Treatment Program: Client Workbook* (New York: Oxford University Press, 2005). Originally described in Michael W. Otto, "Stories and Metaphors in Cognitive-Behavior Therapy," *Cognitive-Behavioral Practice* 7, no. 2 (2000), pp. 166–172.

15. Aaron T. Beck, Cognitive Therapy and the Emotional Disorders (Madison, CT: International Universities Press, Inc., 1975).

Step 6. Manage Your Emotions

1. Russell A. Barkley and Mariellen Fischer, "The Unique Contribution of Emotional Impulsiveness to Impairment in Major Life Activities

in Hyperactive Children as Adults," *Journal of the American Academy of Child and Adolescent Psychiatry* 49, no. 5 (May 2010): 503–513.

2. Paul Ekman, *Emotions Revealed: Recognizing Faces and Feelings to Improve Communication and Emotional Life* (New York: Times Books, 2003).

3. This exercise is adapted from Jon Kabat-Zinn's MBSR program in *Full Catastrophe Living: Using the Wisdom of Your Body and Mind to Face Stress, Pain, and Illness* (New York: Delacorte Press, 1990).

4. Marsha M. Linehan, *Skills Training Manual for Treating Borderline Personality Disorder* (New York: Guilford, 1993).

5. Mark R. Leary et al., "Self-Compassion and Reactions to Unpleasant Self-Relevant Events: The Implications of Treating Oneself Kindly," *Journal of Personality and Social Psychology* 92, no. 5 (2007): 887–904.

6. Barbara Fredrickson, "The Value of Positive Emotions," *American Scientist* 91, no. 4 (July–August 2003): 330–335.

7. Robert A. Emmons, *Thanks! How the New Science of Gratitude Can Make You Happier* (Boston: Houghton Mifflin, 2007).

8. Deborah D. Danner, David A. Snowdon, and Wallace V. Friesen, "Positive Emotions in Early Life and Longevity: Findings from the Nun Study," *Journal of Personality and Social Psychology* 80, no. 5 (2001): 804–813.

9. The HUMAINE Emotion Annotation and Representation Language (EARL). The emotion categories are from http://emotion-research.net/projects/humaine/earl/proposal#Categories. See E. Douglas-Cowie et al., "The HUMAINE Database: Addressing the Collection and Annotation of Naturalistic and Induced Emotional Data," in *Proceedings of the Affective Computing and Intelligent Interaction* (Lisbon, Portugal, 2007), pp. 488–500. Retreived from http://dx.doi.org/10.1007/978-3-540-74889-2_43.

Step 7. Communicate Skillfully

1. Philip Shaw et al., "Attention-Deficit/Hyperactivity Disorder Is Characterized by a Delay in Cortical Maturation," *PNAS* 104, no. 49 (December 2007): 19649–19654.

Step 8. Slow Down to Be More Effective

1. Steven Hayes, *Get Out of Your Mind and Into Your Life: The New Acceptance and Commitment Therapy* (Oakland, Calif.: New Harbinger, 2005).

2. Mary Pipher, *Reviving Ophelia: Saving the Selves of Adolescent Girls* (New York: Ballantine, 1995), 157.

3. Russell A. Barkley, Keven R. Murphy, and Tracie Bush, "Time

Perception and Reproduction in Young Adults with Attention Deficit Hyperactivity Disorder," *Neuropsychology* 15, no. 3 (July 2001): 351–360; and Eve M. Valera et al., "Neural Substrates of Impaired Sensorimotor Timing in Adult Attention-Deficit/Hyperactivity Disorder," *Biological Psychiatry* 68, no. 4 (August 2010): 359–367.

Chapter 4. Putting It All Together

1. See, for example, the website of the Association for Mindfulness in Education, at http://www.mindfuleducation.org/about.html.

ADHD Symptoms Checklist

1. The World Health Organization Adult ADHD Self-Report Scale (ASRS-v1.1) Symptom Checklist. See R. C. Kessler et al., "The World Health Organization Adult ADHD Self-Report Scale (ASRS): A Short Screening Scale for Use in the General Population," in *Psychological Medicine* 35 no. 2 (Feb. 2005): 245–256.

Index

acceptance, 15, 119. *See also* RAIN
    practice
Acceptance Commitment Therapy
    (ACT), 176
acting with awareness, 15
action(s), 133–35
    avoidance of, 170
    choice about your, 1
    mindfulness of, 170–71
    principles in using mindfulness
        with, 171–74
    strategies for getting things
        done, 174–75
        choosing a task, 175–79
        doing a task, 184–87
        finishing the task, 188–89
        starting a task, 179–84
ADHD (attention deficit
    hyperactivity disorder)
    "being in the moment" and,
        21–22
    as deficit in attention regulation,
        31–32
    observing one's own patterns in,
        49–50

symptoms, 2–3
terminology, 1–2
treating self-regulation
    difficulties in, 29–31
See also specific topics
ADHD life, living with and loving
    your, 200–201
ADHD mind, 110–12
ADHD Symptoms Checklist,
    206–8
aerobic exercise, 103
"aha!" moment
    famous, 118
    making room for the, 117–18
alert arousal, 56
alerting, 56
all-or-nothing thinking, 123–25
allowing, 21
anxiety, witnessing, 136
appreciation of self, 141, 167
assumptions, making, 124–25
attention
    in ADHD life, 58
    "bottom-up" vs. "top-down," 58
    compared with a flashlight, 57

attention (*continued*)
  focused vs. open, 19
  mindfulness and, 19, 59–60
  nature of, 11
  paying, 11–12
  paying attention to one's, 6
  to the present moment, 17–18
  to the right thing at the right
    time, 58
  science of, 56–58
  shapes our lives, 11–12
  training, 12
  See also specific topics
attention blink, 41
attention control, mindfulness
    and, 32–33
attention deficit hyperactivity
    disorder. *See* ADHD
attention networks, 56–58
attention regulation
  vs. attention, 31
  See also self-regulation
automatic pilot (autopilot), 12–14,
    56
  can work for or against us, 14
  combining mindfulness and,
    189–90
automatic response, 1
awareness
  about one's actions, 1
  directing and anchoring,
    80–88
  foreground vs. background, 85
  mindful (*see* mindfulness)
  mindfulness as "dropping into,"
    59
  mindfulness as practice of, 22
  training, 12

Barkley, Russell, 24, 28, 50, 129
belly, breath in the, 71–72

Bertin, Mark, 165
black-and-white thinking, 123–25
blaming others or oneself, 123–24
body
  emotions arising in, 131
  learning and listening to the, 90
  See also movement; sensations
body scan, 91–95
  in daily life, 96
boredom in sitting practice, 76–77
brain, training. *See* neuroplasticity
breath, 69, 71, 78–79, 165–66
  importance of the, 70
  is always in the present, 70
  is the door to changing mind-
    body state, 70
  setting the intention to notice
    one's, 84
  staying with and returning to
    the, 73, 76
"Breathing In, I Am Like . . .",
    181–82
Brown, Kirk, 36

calm focus, 172–73
Carney, Dana, 100
CBT. *See* cognitive behavioral
    therapy
chest, breath in the, 71
children, mindfulness for, 198–99
Chödrön, Pema 48
choice regarding one's actions, 1
choiceless awareness. *See* "Mindful
    Presence"
Christoff, Kalina, 116
closing tasks, 188
clumsiness, ADHD and, 96–97
coaching, 29, 185
cognitive behavioral therapy
    (CBT), 29, 122, 123–25, 185
communication

observing one's own, 156–58
in relationships, 160
communication pitfalls, ADHD
    and, 154–56
compassion, 145–46
compassionate communication. *See*
    nonviolent communication
compassionate thinking,
    developing, 122–23
computer-based training, 12, 29
concentration vs. open attention
    and awareness, 19–20
conflict attention, 57
criticism, sensitivity to, 158–60
curiosity, 15, 17–18

dancing meditation, 101–2
Davidson, Richard, 37–38
daydreaming
    knowing that one is, 117
    mindful, 115–17
    science of, 116
delayed gratification, 23
describing with awareness, 15
Dialectical Behavioral Therapy
    (DBT), 17, 30, 119,
    144–45
discernment, 20
distractions, 144
    coming back after, 185
    paying attention despite, 57
    in sitting practice, 76
divided attention, 58
doubting thoughts, 76–77

emotion regulation, 128
    mindfulness and, 34–36
    See also self-regulation
emotion regulation problems and
    communication pitfalls, 156

emotional control, 28
emotional reactions, 131–36
emotions, 128, 166–67
    in ADHD, 129–30
    arise in mind and body, 131
    difficult, 76
        mindfulness of, 136, 153
        willingness to experience,
            147–49
    as dynamic process, 131
    insights into, 130–32
    labeling, 152
    noticing, 183–84
    (over)identification vs.
        non-identification/dis-
        identification with, 48, 105,
        137–39, 166, 197 (*see also*
        RAIN practice)
    positive, 149–51
    principles of and insights into,
        130–31
    "refractory period," 131
    refraining from acting on,
        149
    responding to, 140–41
    words for labeling, 130–31
empathy in relationships affected
    by ADHD, developing,
    162–64
executive functions (EFs), 27–31
    and communication pitfalls,
        155
    examples of, 28
    self-regulation and, 27–29
exercise, physical, 30, 44, 103
experiential avoidance, 136

Farb, Norman, 112
feelings. *See* emotions
finishing tasks, 188
fish oil, 30

focus, 20, 59. *See also*
  concentration vs. open
  attention and awareness
focused attention, 19
focusing on one thing at a time,
  185
foreground and background
  awareness, 60, 85
forgiveness, 147

habits
  creating good, 189–90
  training good, 190–91
habitual response, 1
"hate-it-but-do-it center" of the
  mind, 183
Hayes, Steven, 176
hearing, 62
  setting the intention to notice
  sounds, 83
  See also listening; senses
Hölzel, Britta, 42

images, 115, 167, 173
impulse control, 28. *See also*
  delayed gratification
impulsiveness
  and communication pitfalls,
  155
  emotional, 129
intention, matching attention
  with, 83–85
involuntary ("bottom-up")
  attention, 58

Jha, Amishi, 32, 34
judgmental thinking, 119–22
  vs. "anything goes,"
  204–5

vs. nonjudgmental attitude,
  14–15, 65–66
judgmental thoughts
  counting, 120–21
  neutralizing strong and painful,
  121
  observing, 120–21

Kabat-Zinn, Jon, 16–17, 37
Kaiser-Greenland, Susan, 199
Kuyken, Willem, 35

labeling thoughts and feelings,
  47–49
Lazar, Sarah, 41
learning, using body to enhance,
  104
learning styles, 104
Lehnhoff, John, 183
letting go, 20–21
Linnehan, Marsha, 119
listening
  fully, 161
  mindful, 160–61, 166
  See also hearing
lists, making, 184–85
"Loving-Kindness Meditation,"
  141–43
loving-kindness to self, extending,
  167

MacLean, Katherine, 32–33
magnifying, 124
marshmallow test, 23
massage, 103–4
medications for ADHD, 29
  vs. meditation, 202
  mindfulness practice and,
  202–3

meditation, 18, 202, 203
    concentration and open
        attention exercises, 19–20
    difficulties in sitting practice,
        73–77
    mindfulness and, 19, 203, 204
    posture, 45
    purposes, 204
    spiritual practice and, 203
    See also Transcendental
        Meditation
memory, 33–34
mental training compared with
    physical training, 44
mind-body connection, 100–101,
    103
mind traps, ADHD, 123–25
mindful awareness. *See*
    mindfulness
Mindful Awareness Practices
    (MAPs), 6
"Mindful Breathing," 72–73
mindful breathing in daily life,
    78–79. *See also* breath
"Mindful Listening and Speaking,"
    160–61
"Mindful Movement," 97–98
"Mindful Presence," 165–67
mindful state of mind, 17
"Mindful Walking," 98–99
mindfulness
    ADHD and, 21, 31–38
    benefits of, 32–35, 37–39
    in daily life, 64–65, 194–98 (*see
        also* mindfulness practice:
        informal)
    definition and nature of, 3–5,
        12, 14–16, 20, 22, 55, 59,
        66
    dual nature of, 20
    facets of, 15, 59
    key aspects of, 17–18

as playful practice, 43
spontaneous vs. trained,
    16–17
three anchors of, 85–87
trait/dispositional, 15, 36
See also specific topics
Mindfulness-Based Cognitive
    Therapy (MBCT), 35
Mindfulness-Based Stress
    Reduction (MBSR), 16–17,
    37, 42
"Mindfulness of Sound, Breath,
    and Body," 83–85
mindfulness practice
    alone vs. with others, 46–47
    difficulties in, 46, 47, 73
    formal, 44–47, 68. *See also end of
        each step*
    informal, 44, 47 (*see also*
        mindfulness: in daily life)
    length, 47
    location of, 45–47
    reminders for, 66–67
    tips on, 45–47
minimizing, 124
Mischel, Walter, 23–24
monitoring
    attention, 59
    open, 32, 33
    See also self-monitoring
motivation, finding and jump-
    starting your, 180–82
"Mountain Meditation,"
    173–74
movement (body), 97–98,
    101–2
movement of attention and
    awareness, 56–57, 81–82
multitasking with mindfulness,
    185–86
music, 182
    and meditation, 81–83

neurofeedback, 29
neuroplasticity, 39–40
    examples of, 40
    meditation as stimulating
        healthy, 41–42
noise, 76. *See also* distractions
nonjudgment. *See* judgmental
        thinking
nonreactiveness, 15
nonviolent communication (NVC),
        161–62
nostrils, breath in the, 71

observing (one's reactions)
    with awareness, 15
    nonjudgmentally, 14–15, 65–66,
        204–5
    See also mindfulness
obvious, not seeing the, 124–25
open attention, 19
open monitoring, 32, 33
openness, 15, 17–18
organizing, 28, 184
orienting, 56–57
Orlov, Melissa, 164

pain, 104–6
    vs. suffering, 105
parenting, ADHD and, 164–65
patience, 146–47
pausing, 55–56, 171, 187
Pera, Gina, 164
planning, 28
polarized thinking, 123–25
positive psychology, science of, 150
Posner, Michael, 56–57
posture during mindfulness
        practice, 45, 47
preoccupied mind and sitting
        practice, 76

present-moment experience, 16,
        66
    attention to, 17–18
    pausing and shifting attention
        to, 55–56
    remembering to focus on, 22, 66
    See also specific topics
prioritizing, 28, 184–85
procrastination, 26, 170–71
psychology, mindfulness, and
        spirituality, 199

RAIN practice, 137–39
reinforcement, positive, 189
relationships
    affected by ADHD, 162–64
    mindfulness and, 38–39
relaxation, muscle, 103–4
relaxation response, breath as
        inducing, 70
religion and mindfulness, 203
remembering
    to focus on present moment,
        22, 66
    mindfulness as practice of, 22,
        66
restlessness, 105, 107
    in sitting practice, 74–75
    tips on working with, 107–8
rigid thinking, 125
Rosenberg, Marshall, 161–62
rules-based thinking vs. lack of
        rules, 125
Ryan, Richard, 36

Schooler, Jonathan, 116
seeing, 62. *See also* senses
selective attention, 58
self-appreciation, 141, 167
self-coaching, mindful, 174

self-compassion vs. self-esteem, 146
self-control. *See* self-regulation
self-judgmental thoughts
  being too hard on yourself, 121–22
  neutralizing strong and painful, 121
  See also judgmental thoughts
self-monitoring, 28
self-perception, ADHD and, 111–12
self-regulation, 3, 23–24
  ADHD as disorder of, 24
  executive functions and, 27–29
  nature of, 24, 25
  strategies/approaches to, 24–27
  See also emotion regulation
self-regulation difficulties in ADHD, treating, 29–31
self-regulation strength, 24
self-transcendence, 21
sensations, body, 83, 91, 133–35, 166
  setting the intention to notice, 84–85
  working with difficult, 104–5
senses
  direct experience of the, 61
  rediscovering the, 60–62
  tuning in to the, 62–63
sensory input and ADHD, 63–64
sensory overload, 63–64
sensory processing difficulties, 64
Serenity Prayer, 119
"Shaking and Dancing Meditation," 101–2
Siegel, Dan, 38
Singh, Nirbay, 30, 36, 39
sitting practice
  difficulties in, 73–77

See also meditation
Slagter, Heleen, 41
sleepiness in sitting practice, 74–75
Smalley, Susan, 21
smelling, 62–63. *See also* senses
smile, "soft," 103
speaking with awareness, 160–61
spirituality, psychology, and mindfulness, 199
STOP practice, 86–87, 126
  using it with tasks, 171–72
  as visual reminder, 87–88
  as you talk, 157–58
stress, 36–38
suffering. *See* pain
supportive thinking, developing, 122–23
surrender, 20–21
sustained attention, 58

tai chi, 31
Tang, Yi-Yuan, 41–42
tasks
  managing, 28
  See also action(s)
tasting, 63. *See also* senses
therapies that use mindfulness exercises, 17. *See also specific therapies*
thinking, 110
  mindfulness of, 112
  mindfulness of unhelpful, 118–19
  watching one's thinking under a tree, 114–15
thoughts, 110, 133–35, 167
  dealing with uncomfortable, 76, 118
  sensing the space in between one's, 113

time management, 28, 191–92
touching, 63. *See also* senses
Transcendental Meditation (TM),
    19, 31
  vs. mindfulness, 18–21
transitioning out of tasks, 188–89

UCLA Mindful Awareness
    Research Center, 6, 203
Uliando, Anna, 7, 30
uncomfortable thoughts or
    feelings, 76

values, clarifying your, 176–79
values worksheet, 177–79
van der Oord, Saskia, 30–31
vigilance, 56
Vipassana, 19. *See also* meditation
visual attention and awareness,
    playing with, 59–60

visualizations, 115
voluntary ("top-down") attention,
    58

walking, mindful, 98–99
Wallace, Alan, 32–33
wandering mind, 73–74. *See also*
    specific topics
willpower, 24
witnessing perspective, 6, 35, 48,
    112, 114, 136. *See also specific*
    topics
working memory, 28, 33

yoga, 31, 98

"zone," being in the, 82

About the Author

Dr. Lidia Zylowska is one of the cofounders of the UCLA Mindful Awareness Research Center, where she serves as assistant clinical professor. She is a board-certified psychiatrist specializing in adult psychiatry, mindfulness-based therapy, and adult ADHD.

In 2003, Dr. Zylowska was awarded the UCLA Robert Wood Johnson Clinical Scholars Program Fellowship during which, in collaboration with the UCLA Center for Neurobehavioral Genetics, she developed Mindful Awareness Program for ADHD: a mindfulness-based training in attention self-regulation.

Dr. Zylowska's private practice is located in West Los Angeles. For more information, including a schedule of workshops and other events, please visit www.lidiazylowska.com.

CD Track List

1. Introduction (0:32)
2. Mindful Breathing (6:06)
3. Sound, Breath, and Body (11:41)
4. Body Scan (12:01)
5. Mindful Walking (4:49)
6. Mind Like a Sky (7:47)
7. RAIN (6:49)
8. Loving Kindness (7:25)
9. Mindful Presence (10:08)